ORAL AND MAXILLOFACIAL IMAGING TECHNIQUES

ORAL AND MAXILLOFACIAL IMAGING TECHNIQUES

SHIVLAL M RAWLANI
BDS MDS (Oral Medicine and Radiology)
Associate Professor and Head
Department of Dentistry
Mahatma Gandhi Institute of Medical Sciences
Sevagram, Wardha, Maharashtra, India

Co-author
SHOBHA S RAWLANI
MBBS MS (Anatomy)
Professor and Head
Department of Anatomy
Dr Panjabrao Deshmukh Memorial Medical College
Amravati, Maharashtra, India

Forewords
VEDPRAKASH MISHRA
P NARANG

JAYPEE

JAYPEE BROTHERS MEDICAL PUBLISHERS (P) LTD
New Delhi • London • Philadelphia • Panama

Jaypee Brothers Medical Publishers (P) Ltd

Headquarters
Jaypee Brothers Medical Publishers (P) Ltd
4838/24, Ansari Road, Daryaganj
New Delhi 110 002, India
Phone: +91-11-43574357
Fax: +91-11-43574314
Email: jaypee@jaypeebrothers.com

Overseas Offices

J.P. Medical Ltd
83, Victoria Street, London
SW1H 0HW (UK)
Phone: +44-2031708910
Fax: +02-03-0086180
Email: info@jpmedpub.com

Jaypee-Highlights Medical Publishers Inc.
City of Knowledge, Bld. 237, Clayton
Panama City, Panama
Phone: +507-301-0496
Fax: +507-301-0499
Email: cservice@jphmedical.com

Jaypee Medical Inc.
The Bourse
111 South Independence Mall East
Suite 835, Philadelphia, PA 19106, USA
Phone: + 267-519-9789
Email: joe.rusko@jaypeebrothers.com

Jaypee Brothers Medical Publishers (P) Ltd
17/1-B Babar Road, Block-B, Shaymali
Mohammadpur, Dhaka-1207
Bangladesh
Mobile: +08801912003485
Email: jaypeedhaka@gmail.com

Jaypee Brothers Medical Publishers (P) Ltd
Bhotahity, Kathmandu, Nepal
Phone: +977-9741283608
Email: kathmandu@jaypeebrothers.com

Website: www.jaypeebrothers.com
Website: www.jaypeedigital.com

Inquiries for bulk sales may be solicited at: jaypee@jaypeebrothers.com

Oral and Maxillofacial Imaging Techniques

First Edition: **2014**

ISBN: 978-93-5090-846-4

Printed at Rajkamal Electric Press, Plot No. 2, Phase-IV, Kundli, Haryana.

Dedicated to

Our Beloved Parents
Mihomal H Rawlani
Smt Krishnabai M Rawlani
and
Our Children
Sudhir Rawlani
Sujata Rawlani

Foreword

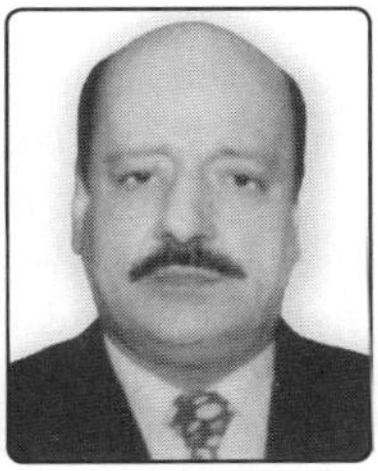

The initiative and the effort diligently articulated by Dr Shivlal M Rawlani, an Ex-Senior Faculty Member in the Department of Oral Medicine and Radiology at Sharad Pawar Dental College, Sawangi (Meghe), Wardha, Maharashtra, India, a constituent unit of Datta Meghe Institute of Medical Sciences (Deemed University), Nagpur, Maharashtra in bringing out a book titled *Oral and Maxillofacial Imaging Techniques* is exemplary at one end and genuinely praiseworthy at the other.

It is indeed an effort to compile all the relevant intellectual inputs on a significantly vital area and render them in such a free flowing manner, so that it is easy to understand, decipher, and assimilate by the learner, teacher, a professional and otherwise a reader as well.

This has been singularly achieved by the author by virtue of his writings, which are in easy textual format and are appropriately syntaxed, so as to render the desired grasp and sought after understanding of the subject in a handy but yet in an immaculate manner, which turns out to be the unique feature of this authorship, which makes it look and feel different from the other available reading material on the subject as of now.

It is, indeed, a fact that maxillofacial region is not only anatomically complex region of the human body, in as much as it has several elements and organs from the different systems that get affected by several pathological processes. The anatomical complexity makes it all the more difficult to diagnose the affecting pathologies exclusively on the basis of clinical skills. It is for this very reason, the aiding diagnostic tools turn out to be of huge significance and relevance of which 'Diagnostic Imaging' has earned a central place in evaluation of this region. Radiography *per se* has turned out to be one of the most significant diagnostic tools over a period of time, and now it is in routine usage for more than one reason if relevant.

It is an evident reality that for a very long time, the radiography film was the long and yet a very pertinent modality in the domain of diagnostic imaging. But the advent of technology at a very rapid pace in the context of electronic era has made a sea change, whereby several specialized techniques and instrumentations stand incorporated in the operational arena, which has now made it multifaceted.

The author has brought out all the imaging techniques in usage in a very deserving, appropriate, and chronologically lucid manner. The chapters' sequence vividly brings out the continuum from conventional radiography of yesteryears to the present-day magnetic imaging techniques with due incorporation of tomogrophy, computed tomography, sialography, sialoscopy, arthrography, arthroscopy, temporomandibular junction (TMJ) imaging, subtraction radiography, radiovisiography, implant radiology, teleradiography, photostimulable phosphor radiography collectively grouped under the ionizing imaging techniques and digital radiography, and ultrasonography as nonionizing imaging techniques in between.

Each of the radioimaging techniques has been dealt with in all the need-based relevant details that include description of the technique, their indications, contraindications, advantages, and limitations as well. As a matter of fact, the extent of coverage worked out by the author is indeed very vast but has been so well capsulated that it makes it poignantly a very interesting reading and learning material, as well.

I am sure that this elegant piece of scientific literature embodied in the book format by the author will make every user feel that he/she could avail all that he/she desired, needed, and expected out of it. I have no hesitation in putting on record my appreciation for the effort undertaken by the author in terms of a loud statement that he has generated a 'satiety center' for quenching the inquisitional thirst' in the domain of radioimaging techniques in dentistry.

Vedprakash Mishra MD
Pro-Chancellor
Datta Meghe Institute of Medical Sciences
(Deemed University)
Nagpur, Maharashtra, India

Foreword

What would it be like in a radiologist's shoes? To spend most of my day dealing with images of people: plain black-and-white X-ray images, or speckled images caused by sound waves bouncing off organs, or images caused by dyes outlining arteries and veins, or contrast medium filling loops of bowel, or images reconstructed by computers into cross-sections of the body—all without speaking to a patient.

— My Own Country, Abraham Verghese, 1994

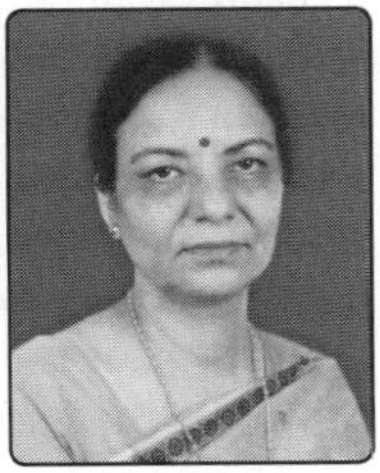

Roentgen Wilhelm Conard was experimenting with the conduction of electricity in a vacuum tube when he noticed a strange fluorescence on a barium screen lying nearby. Further experiments indicated that the fluorescence was created by some invisible rays from the tube. These rays could also pass through substances that ordinary light could not penetrate and they could also affect the photographic film. Roentgen named these rays as X-rays, and they are also often called after the name of the discoverer. This occurred in 1895, and Roentgen received the world's first Nobel Prize in Physics in 1901.

Roentgen even in his remotest dream could not have ever imagined the revolution that his discovery was likely to bring about in the next hundred years not only in its fundamental application of physics but also in medical science. If any discovery has actually promoted the path of disease diagnosis in medicine by affecting the majority patients, it is the discovery of X-rays. Today, the explosive knowledge accumulated over the years has become so intricate and technically complex that it is almost beyond complete comprehension. Conventional radiography has given way to more sensitive modalities, such as the sonography, tomography, and electromagnetic radiography. These advances have also paved the way for intervention radiology, and unlike the statement made by Abraham Verghese quoted above; the radiologists are also now getting a chance to talk to the patients. However, there is a need to present these complexities in a more simple and comprehendible manner particularly for the uninitiated students. The authors, by bringing out this book have addressed these complexities in a simple intelligent manner without compromising with the essence and accuracy. They have stuck to their belief that any radiologists, whether in dentistry or in medicine, can only be good in interpreting the images if he/she understands the fundamental physics and basic principles of the equipment that he/she is using. Moreover, the basic principle of any diagnostic laboratory or unit is that the medical person venturing to interpret the results must first himself be a good technician. A medical radiologist must, along with other things, have full knowledge of technical details, such as positioning of the patient, amount and time of exposure, developing of films, nature of the dyes and contrasts used, and then only will he/she be able to photograph the correct target site. With the advent of nuclear medicine, radiology has entered into yet another arena of diagnosis giving the relevant definitions and the uses of positron emission tomography (PET), single-photon emission computed tomography (SPECT), and other techniques. The very fact that the authors have restricted to a small portion, i.e. maxillofacial imaging, is in itself an indicator that radioimaging and interpretation of every part has become a science in itself. Writing a story book or a novel depends on author's ability to imagine and fantasize. Authoring a technical and a professional volume requires knowledge, experience, and expertise.

Dr Shivlal M Rawlani with his vast experience as a teacher and community worker, along with Dr Shobha S Rawlani, has understood the difficulties of the budding radiologists and has, therefore, brought out this book that would be useful not only to students of dentistry but also to aspiring radiologists in medical schools.

The book is clinically relevant and practical to use. The chapters are straightforward, well illustrated, and the basics have been simplified, making the text easily understandable. I am sure that every individual who reads the book would like to possess it.

P Narang MD
Dr BC Roy Awardee
Secretary
Kasturba Health Society
Director Professor
Department of Microbiology
Mahatma Gandhi Institute of Medical Sciences
Sevagram, Wardha, Maharashtra, India

Preface

The book provides the basic knowledge of oral and maxillofacial imaging techniques used in dentistry, which is important for every student of dental and medical faculty and also preparing for entrance examination. The student undergoing postgraduation in Oral Medicine and Radiology, and Oral and Maxillofacial Surgery will also find this book very beneficial.

In this book, attempt has been made to introduce most of imaging techniques being used in dentistry under one platform in simple language, which include brief history, clinical implication, indications, contraindications, advantages, disadvantages, and complications of every technique.

As this is the first edition of the book, there may be few mistakes/errors in text, we will be very thankful to the teachers and the students for sending suggestions and drawing attention towards the errors.

Shivlal M Rawlani
Shobha S Rawlani

Acknowledgments

I would like to thank:

- My guide and mentor Dr Mukta B Motwani, Professor and Head, Department of Oral Medicine and Radiology, VSPM Dental College, Nagpur, for his encouragement and moral support
- Dr Shirish Degwekar, Professor and Head, Department of Oral Medicine and Radiology, Sarad Pawar Dental College, Sawangi (Meghe), Wardha, for his strong encouragement and guidance
- Dr Rahul Bhowate, Professor, Department of Oral Medicine and Radiology, Sarad Pawar Dental College, Sawangi (Meghe), Wardha, for his valuable suggestions and support
- Dr Rajiv Borle, Registrar, Datta Meghe Institute of Medical Sciences (Deemed University), for his strong encouragement and guidance
- Dr Ashok Pakhan, Dean, Sharad Pawar Dental College, Sawangi, Wardha, for his valuable suggestions and cooperation
- Mr Dirubhai Mehta, President, Kasturba Health Society, Mahatma Gandhi Institute of Medical Sciences, Sevagram, for his valuable suggestions and cooperation
- Dr P Narang, Secretary, Kasturba Health Society, Mahatma Gandhi Institute of Medical Sciences, Sevagram, for her appreciable suggestions
- Dr BS Garge, Dean, Kasturba Health Society, Mahatma Gandhi Institute of Medical Sciences, Sevagram, for his valuable suggestions and cooperation
- Dr Panjab Wanjari, Dean, Modern Dental College, Indore, for his valuable suggestions and cooperation
- Dr Zade, Dean, Chhattisgarh Dental College and Research Center, Rajnandgaon, for his valuable suggestions and cooperation
- Dr Lokwani, Vice Chancellor, Madhya Pradesh Health University, for his strong encouragement and guidance
- Dr Krishnmohan, Dean, Sibar Dental Institute and Research Center, Guntur, for his valuable suggestions and advice
- Dr Atul Tayde, Professor and Head, Department of Radiology, Mahatma Gandhi Institute of Medical Sciences, Sevagram, for his valuable suggestions and cooperation
- Dr Shyam Chaudhari, for his support and encouragement

- Shri Jitendar P Vij (Group Chairman), Mr Ankit Vij (Managing Director) and Mr Tarun Duneja (Director-Publishing) of M/s Jaypee Brothers Medical Publishers (P) Ltd, New Delhi, India, for accepting my project and publishing the book
- My special thanks to my dear friends and colleagues, Dr Atul Indurkar, Dr Anil Ghom, Dr Ranjit Patil, Dr Sathwane, Dr Modi, Dr Vinod Patni, Dr Umargi, Dr Dinkar, Dr Bhashkar Patle, Dr Pankaj Banode, Dr Kailash Singhaniya, Dr Ranjit Kamble, Dr Baloor, Dr BK Motwani, Dr Bhongade, Dr Niranjan Naidu, Dr Dhirwani, Dr Vidhya Lohe, Dr Suwarna Dangore, Dr Arti Panchbhai, Dr Ravi Raj, Dr Sarat Gumdupu, Dr Bollanagesh, Dr Ravi Kiran, Dr Sunita Puranic, Dr Deepak Samdhani, Dr Gadhewar, Dr Rajesh Gondhrekar, Dr Adwani, Dr Nita Mishra, Dr Mobin, and Dr Ramnic
- My special thanks to Dr Sunil Mishra and our artist Mr Satish Shingare, for their kind support
- My heartfelt thanks to my wife Dr Shobha S Rawlani, my son Sudhir, and my daughter Sujata whose valuable support has made possible to complete the book. I am also thankful to my dearest Dr Rakhi Chandak, Dr Manoj Chandak, Dr Bharti Adwani, and Dr Sangita Wadhwan
- I am immensely thankful to Dr Rucha Atmaramani and my daughter Dr Sujata Rawlani, for their valuable help in composing and editing the material for this book.

Shivlal M Rawlani

Contents

1 Introduction

INTRODUCTION

The maxillofacial region extends from the base of the skull to the hyoid bone. It is one of the most anatomically complex regions of the body. This area contains elements and organs belonging to a number of different systems that can be affected by various local and systemic pathological processes. Due to anatomical complexity of the maxillofacial region, clinically it is very difficult to examine all the local and systemic pathological processes occurring in the maxillofacial region. To get more accurate diagnosis or information regarding pathology in the maxillofacial region, diagnostic imaging has assumed a central role in the evaluation of this region.

The use of radiograph as a diagnostic tool has become an indispensable routine in dentistry. The presence and extension of many pathologic or abnormal conditions can be traced only by radiograph. In numerous situations, the use of radiographs is also essential during therapy and to follow the progress of treatment effects.

For a long time, radiographic film was the most important medium to achieve the diagnostic image. But with the electronic era, however, more specialized equipments are introduced into different phases of the imaging procedure.

A conventional radiographic image consists of all the arrangement of silver grains in the photographic emulsion. The density of silver grains depends on the intensity of the X-ray beam. When a radiograph is viewed on a light box using transmitted light, the pattern of different densities of the silver grains is transferred to the eyes and perceived as different shades of gray. A structure that lacks sufficient density to attenuate the beam does not appear on the radiograph. If the density of a structure of interest is too low to meet sufficient diagnostic need, the contrast and density can be improved artificially.

With the help of artificial contrast most of the salivary gland lesion and internal derangement of temporomandibular joint (TMJ) can be diagnosed.

The changes first happened in 1980 in dental radiography. Although film based imaging is not yet abandoned completely, digital imaging is now a well-accepted modality.

In digital imaging, instead of silver halide grains, a large number of small light sensitive elements are used to record the image data from the X-ray shadow. To display the image, different shades of gray are produced by the amount of light emitted from the monitor screen. The fundamental difference between conventional radiographic image and digital image is that in radiographic image, the silver grain is randomly dispersed in the emulsion, whereas the electronic elements of a digital sensor are arranged in a regular grid of rows and columns. The quantitative characteristics of the light sensitive elements of the electronic sensor results in gray shades having a discrete value for proper diagnosis.

In maxillofacial region, dental point of view the most commonly affected organs and structures are temporomandibular joint, base of skull, paranasal sinus and salivary glands. Conventional radiographs are routinely used for the examination of this site. However, the overlaps of structures may impair a proper interpretation, because of this 3-dimentional imaging techniques have become increasingly important in diagnostic imaging in the oral and maxillofacial region.

Internal derangement of TMJ may be an important factor in pathogenesis of chronic facial pain and facial dysfunction. For proper evaluation of external and internal changes in TMJ apart from the some conventional radiograph, nowadays many new imaging modalities are used in maxillofacial radiography. Computed tomography (CT), magnetic resonance imaging (MRI), ultrasonography (USG) and computed radiography (CR) are all used. All of them have been developed for making diagnosis, but today they are highly appreciated in the dentistry. As a consequence of this, alternative modalities of investigation like xeroradiography, scintigraphy, etc. were invented and utilized for oral and maxillofacial radiodiagnosis.

Xeroradiography is an electrostatic imaging process in which the image produced by an X-ray beam is recorded on a special plate instead of radiographic film. It is most widespread use is in xeromammography, an accepted diagnostic method in the examination of larynx, tracheo-bronchial tree, lymph nodes, salivary glands, brain, long bone and joints.

Radionuclide salivary imaging (scintigraphy), involves the intravenous injection of radioactive compounds with special affinity for particular tissue and later detection of them by means of external detector and imaging systems. Salivary scintigraphy measures the uptake; concentration and secretion by the salivary glands. Radionuclide imaging, or functional imaging technique are the only means by which physiologic changes that are direct result of biochemical alteration may be assessed.

Angiography, a radiographic procedure carried out by injecting radiopaque dye into vessels and making radiograph. Angiography demonstrates the nature of the vascular derangements, its relationship to the bone defect and associated abnormal arterial and venous vasculature.

Ultrasound is noninvasive, nonionizing imaging technique. Ultrasonography or ultrasound uses sound as sonar does to image structures deep within soft tissue. Ultrasonic scanner uses a transducer to convert electrical energy into high frequency sound waves that pass into the tissue. As the waves strikes, tissues of different densities, some of the vibrational energy is reflected back to the scanning transducer, where the sound waves are converted back to electrical energy. This electrical energy is amplified, enhanced, and displayed on video monitor. It is also good at determining the outlines of structures but not necessarily their contents. Ultrasound is inexpensive, and produces no side effects. Doppler ultrasound is particularly useful in identifying soft tissue vascular lesions.

MRI is the latest noninvasive imaging modality that uses electrical signals generated from the response of hydrogen nuclei (proton) to strong magnetic field and radio waves/radiofrequency pulses to produce an image to allow specialist to explore the inner working of human body, to detect and define the differences between healthy and diseased tissue without the use of X-ray. It enables the radiologist to view, slices of the body cut in different planes increasing the diagnostic ability. MRI can aid in diagnosing TMJ internal derangement.

Conventional radiographic techniques—the advanced radiographic modalities alongwith their indication, contraindications, advantages and disadvantages are discussed in detail.

IMAGING TECHNIQUES FOR MAXILLOFACIAL REGION

Diagnostic imaging has assumed a central role in the evaluation of a host of abnormalities involving the maxillofacial region.

The various imaging techniques for maxillofacial region can be grouped as under:

I. Ionizing Imaging Techniques

- Tomography
- Computed tomography

- Sialography
- Sialoscopy
- Arthrography
- Arthroscopy
- Nuclear medicine
- Temporomandibular joint imaging
- Substraction radiography
- Radiovisiography
- Implant radiology
- Teleradiography
- Photostimulable phosphor radiography.

II. Nonionizing Imaging Techniques

- Ultrasonography
- Magnetic resonance imaging.

2 Conventional Radiography

Ever since the 'dental X-ray pioneers' took the first radiographs of teeth in early1896, radiology has become an integral component in the assessment of the dental patient. The vast majority of radiographs taken in dental practice includes intraoral, but nowadays increasing number of extraoral views are also adviced. The term plain film refers to radiographs made with a stationary X-ray source and film. Plain films depict only the mineralized part but do not reveal non-mineralized cartilage and soft tissues components.

Conventional radiography incorporates intraoral, occlusal and extra-oral radiography. Most anatomical structures and pathologic conditions associated with oral and maxillofacial structures can be imaged using conventional radiography.

INTRAORAL RADIOGRAPHIC TECHNIQUE

The word intraoral radiography means making the radiograph of an oral structure by placing the X-ray film in the oral cavity while X-ray source is outside of the oral cavity. The radiographic image will have five basic characteristics that includes density, contrast, sharpness, distortion and magnification which affects the quality of film and can be controlled by six principles of shadow casting.

1. Radiation source should be as small as possible.
2. The target to object distance should be as long as practically possible.
3. The object to film distance should be as small as possible.
4. The X-ray tube, patient and film should not move during exposure.
5. The film and teeth should be parallel to each other.
6. The central beam should be at right angle to film and object both (Figs 2.1 to 2.4).

Dr Weston A Price in 1904 introduced two techniques for film positioning. There are two basic intraoral radiographic techniques: they are bisecting the angle technique and paralleling technique.

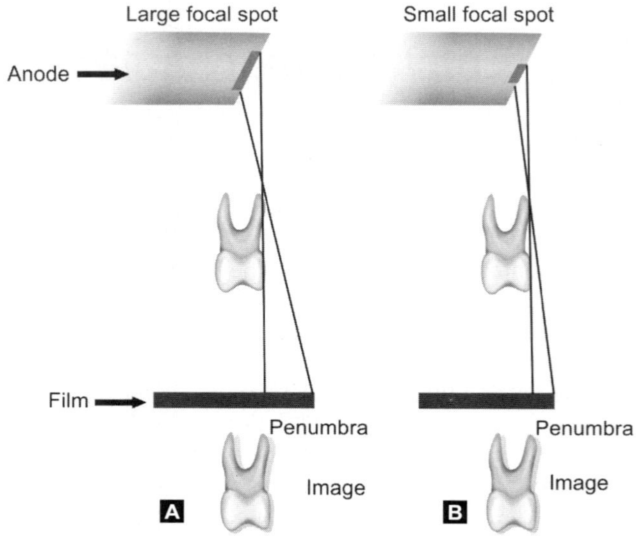

Fig. 2.1: Small focal spot area, the shaper the image, larger the focal spot area—loss of image sharpness

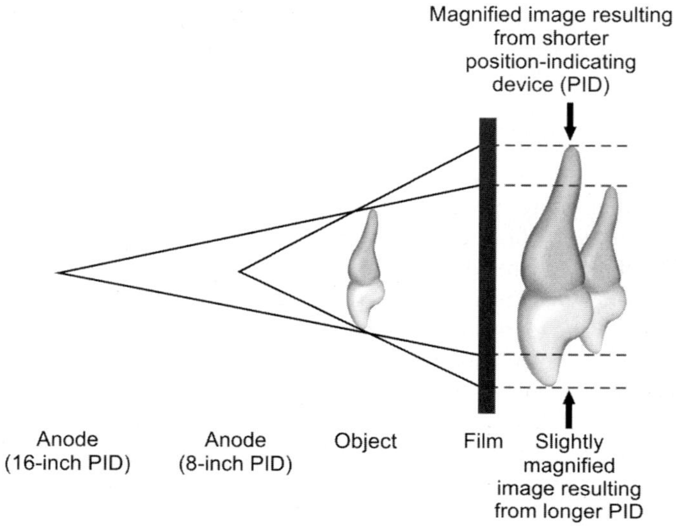

Fig. 2.2: More target film distance reduces magnification

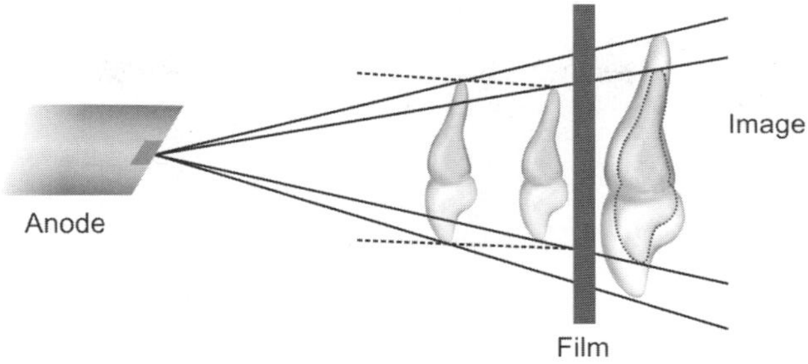

Fig. 2.3: Less the object film distance, less the image enlargement

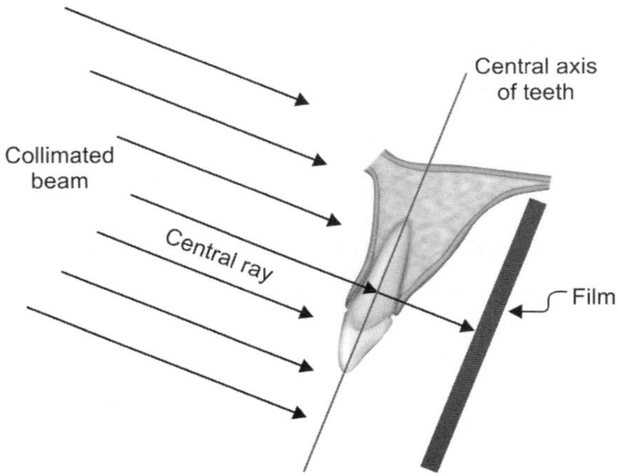

Fig. 2.4: Film and long axis of tooth are parallel to each other and central rays are perpendicular to both

Paralleling Technique

The paralleling technique was developed in 1920 by McCormick. This technique is also known as the Fitzgerald technique, right angle technique, long cone or extended cone technique. The essence of this technique is that the X-ray film is placed parallel to the long axis of the teeth and the central beam of X-ray is directed at right angles to the teeth and film both. To achieve parallelism between the film and the tooth, the film must be placed away from the tooth and toward the middle of the oral cavity (Fig. 2.5).

- The plane of film must be flat and parallel to long axis of tooth
- Film should be placed away from the teeth in the middle of oral cavity except in the mandibular molar region

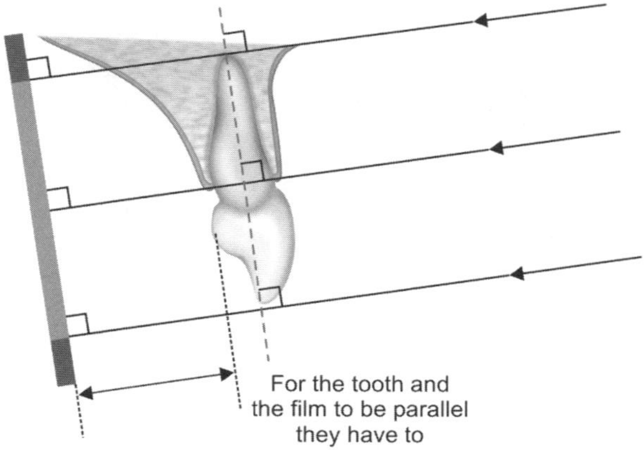

Fig. 2.5: Position of film, tooth and the central beam in paralleling technique

- The cone should be parallel to the film thereby central ray is directed perpendicular to the film
- Target to film distance is increased (16 inches)
- Parallel technique required film holder to place the film parallel to long axis of tooth. The film holders commonly used are Rinn XCP hemostatic with bite block and stable bite block
- Film holder should be selected on the basis of comfort and accuracy of its placement. Film holder with inbuilt centering device are more suitable to assist the centering the X-ray beam.

Placement of X-ray Film

- Exposure side (white) of the film always faces the teeth
- X-ray film is always place vertical for anterior region of jaw
- X-ray film is always place horizontally for posterior region of jaw
- Orientation dot (embossed) is placed occlussally to avoid superimposition of the dot over an apex of teeth (Fig. 2.6)
- When positioning the film holder, always center the film over the area of tooth to be examined
- When positioning the film holder ask the patient to "slowly close" on the bite block. Bite block is stabilized by the teeth and not the lips.

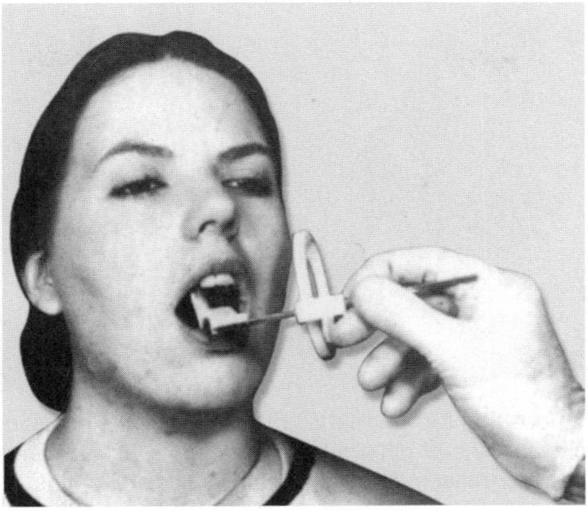

Fig. 2.6: Placement of film in patient mouth by using film holding device with correct side toward the tube head and mounting dot is toward incisal edge

Position of Patient for Paralleling Technique

- Brief information regarding the technique to patient
- Adjust the chair so that patient is positioned upright in the chair
- Secure the lead apron and thyroid collar on the patient
- Locator ring is adjusted such that the indicator rod is just in contact with the patient face, this ensures the correct focal spot to film distance
- The long cone is aligned with the locator ring this automatically sets the vertical and horizontal angulations and help in centering the X-ray beam (Figs 2.7 to 2.10)
- Patients' movement must be avoided during exposure of film.

Advantages

- The paralleling technique produces image that has dimensional accuracy
- There is no overlap of related structures
- The alveolar crest is demonstrated in true relation ship with teeth
- This technique is simple and easy to learn and use
- Less radiation dose to the skin
- Less dose to thyroid gland and lens of eyes
- Duplication of radiograph is possible at different visits and with different operators
- No cone cut

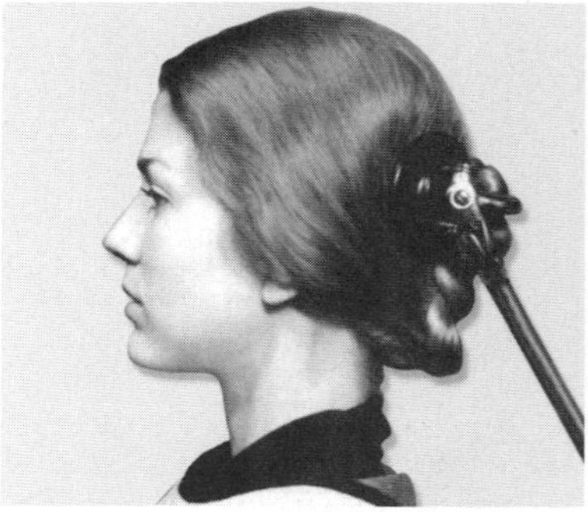

Fig. 2.7: Patients position for maxillary radiograph: Occlusal plane of maxillary teeth or ala-tragus is parallel to floor

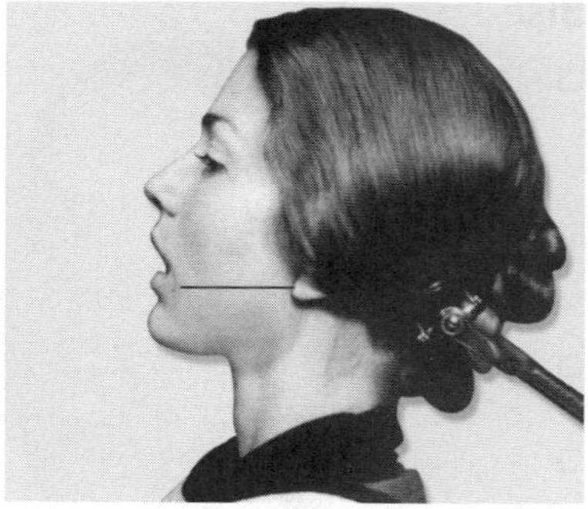

Fig. 2.8: Patients position for mandibular radiograph: Occlusal plane of mandibular teeth is parallel to floor

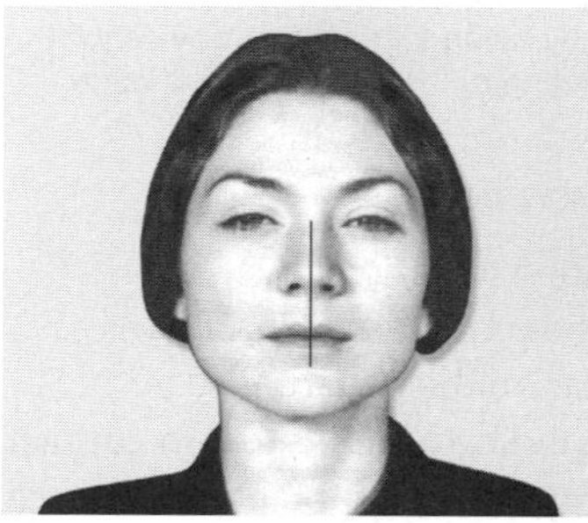

Fig. 2.9: Sagittal plane of head perpendicular to floor

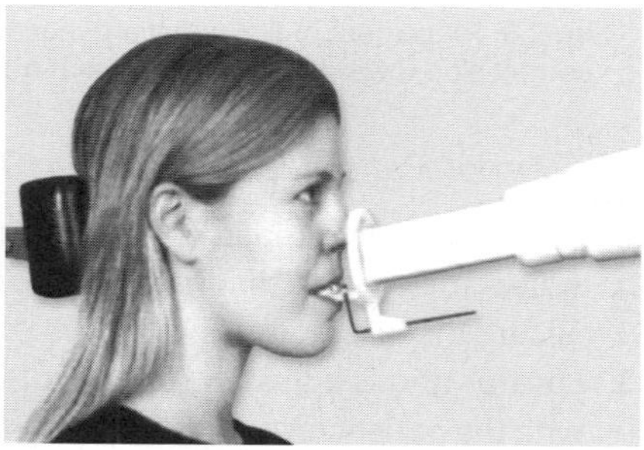

Fig. 2.10: Film position

- The periapical tissues are accurately shown with minimal foreshortening or elongation
- There is decreased secondary radiation.

Disadvantage of Long Cone Technique

- The film holding device is difficult to place and adjust especially in child patients and adults with a small mouth or shallow palate
- Patients discomfort due to impinge of film holding device to the oral soft tissues
- Cannot be performed with short cone technique
- The holder should be autoclave repeatedly
- Requires more exposure time
- Requires more area and it are not so useful in small dental clinics
- Positioning the film in the third molar region can be difficult.

Bisecting Line Angle Technique

- Bisecting line angle technique is also called short cone technique which is based on the rule of isometric. It is based on the principal of geometric theorem of Cieszynski rule, which states that two triangles are equal when they share one common side and have two equal angles. The film is placed as close as possible to the tooth during investigation without bending the film
- The angle formed between the long axis of the tooth and the long axis of the X-ray film packet is assessed
- The X-ray tube head is positioned at right angle to imaginary bisector with the central X-rays beam aimed through the apex of the tooth
- If the X-ray beam is directed right angle to the film the image produced is shorter and if the X-ray beam is directed perpendicular to the long axes of the teeth, then the image is elongated
- The target to object distance in this technique is 8 inches (Figs 2.11 to 2.13).

Patient Position

Patient should sit upright in the chair with well-supported back and head to avoid the movement during exposure.

- While taking maxillary radiograph the head should be positioned downward so that ala-tragus line is parallel to the floor or occlusal plane of maxillary arch is parallel to the floor (Fig. 2.14)

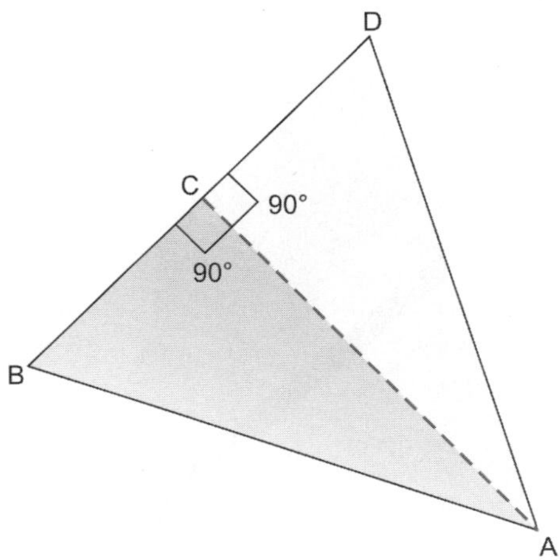

Fig. 2.11: The rule of isometry, two triangles are equal when they have two equal angles and one common side

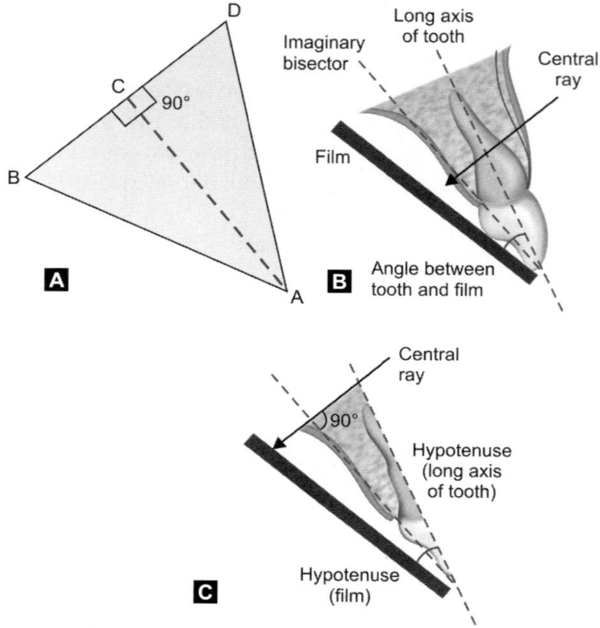

Figs 2.12A to C: (A) Imaginary bisector (AC) divides the angle into two equal angles; (B) Central ray directed perpendicular to the imaginary bisector; (C) Two imaginary triangles that result are equal and congruent

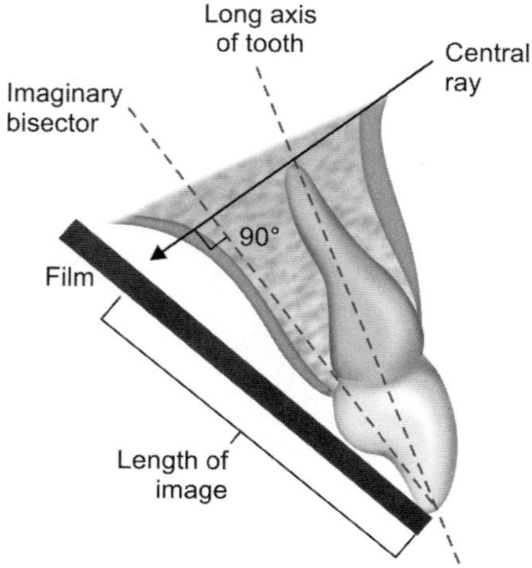

Fig. 2.13: A tooth and its radiographic image will be equal in length when central ray is perpendicular to bisecting line

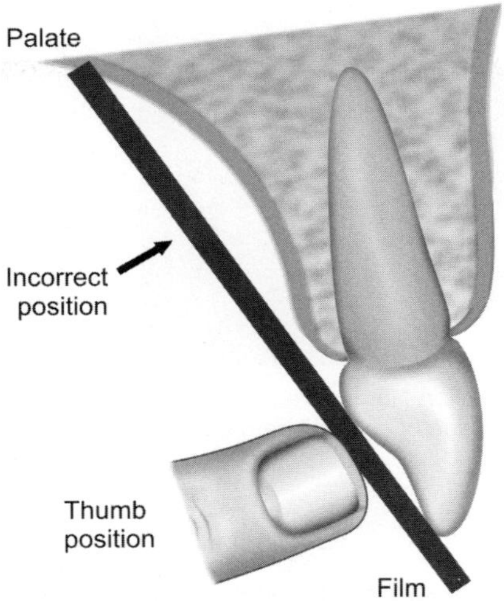

Fig. 2.14: Correct position of thumb to hold the film in patient mouth

- While taking mandibular radiograph chin should be moved upward so that the line drawn from corner of the mouth to the tragus of ear should be parallel to floor or mandibular occlusal plane is parallel to the floor
- Ask the patient to wear lead apron and thyroid collar and remove eye glasses, denture and ornament.

Film Placement

- The exposure surface of the film must face the X-ray beam with embossed dot placed occlussally
- For anterior region of jaw (maxillary and mandibular) long axis of the film should be place vertically
- For posterior regions of jaw (premolar and molar) long axis for the film should be placed horizontally
- About 2 mm of X-ray film packed should extent above the incisal or occlusal edge to ensure that entire tooth appears on the film
- Ask the patient to hold the film gently against the lingnal or palatal surface of the tooth
- Film should be stable in the oral cavity during exposure (Figs 2.15 to 2.18).

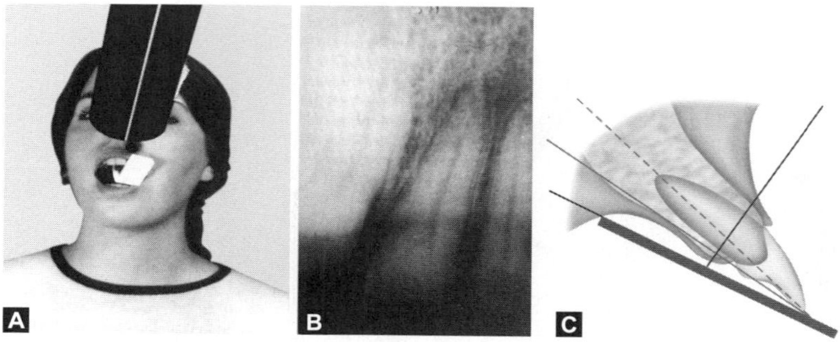

Figs 2.15A to C: Maxillary anterior region: Position of film with the help of PID, direction of central beam and resultant image

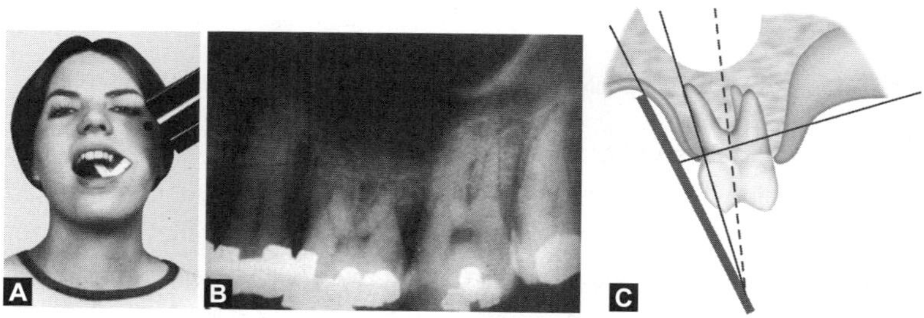

Figs 2.16A to C: Maxillary molar region: Position of film with the help of PID, direction of central beam and resultant image

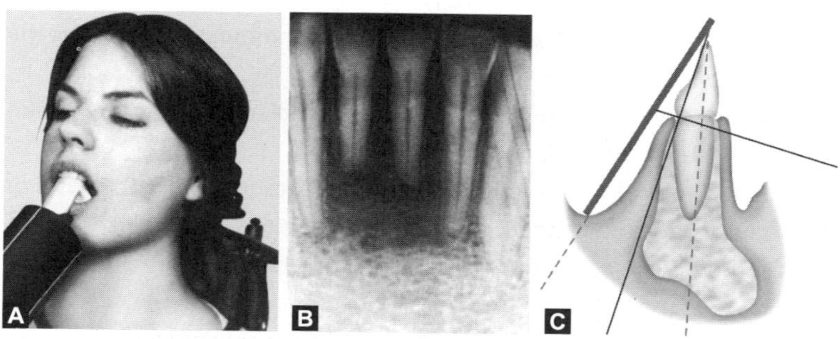

Figs 2.17A to C: Mandibular anterior region: Position of film with the help of PID, direction of central beam and resultant image

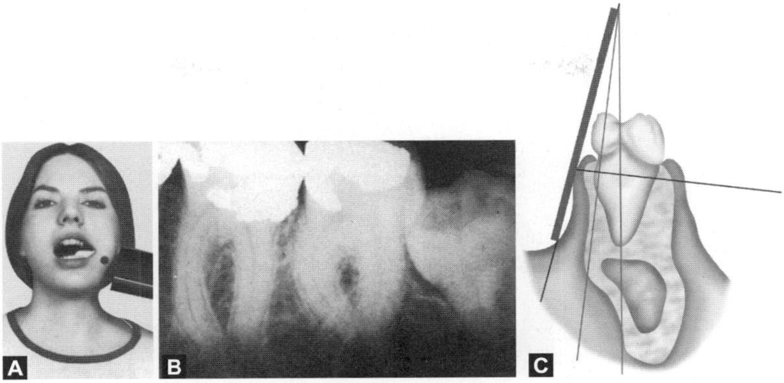

Figs 2.18A to C: Maxillary molar region: Position of film with the help of PID, direction of central beam and resultant image

Vertical Angulation of X-ray Tube Head

Basic principal of X-ray taking is that, the central beam must be perpendicular to object and film both. In bisecting angle technique film is not placed parallel to tooth, hence vertical angulations are used to achieve the central beam perpendicular to imaginary bisector line.

- The angle between the film and teeth depends upon the height of dome of the palate and depth of floor of mouth. The higher the dome less is the angle between the film and teeth, therefore, smaller the vertical angle of central beam
- It is the position of the X-ray tube head in upward and downward direction. If direction of angulation is in downward direction it is called positive vertical angulation and if direction of angulation is in upward direction it is called negative vertical angulation (Fig. 2.19)
- The angle formed by the central ray unit with the occlusal plane determines the vertical angulation of the X-ray beam to the occlusal plane
- Correct vertical angulation results in the image having same length as that of the tooth
- Incorrect vertical angulation results in:

Foreshortening of image is due to, increase in vertical angulation and elongation is due to less vertical angulation (Figs 2.20 and 2.21).

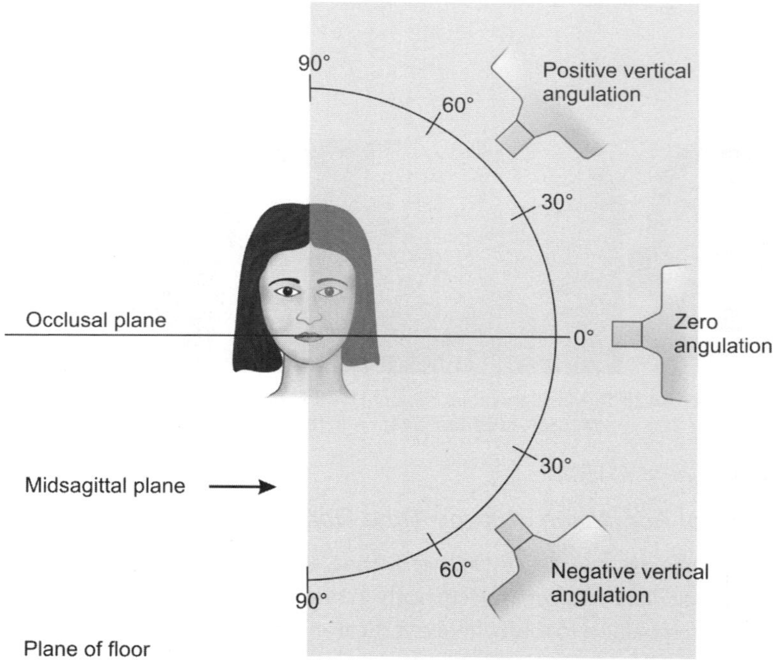

Fig. 2.19: Vertical angulations above the occlusal plane are termed as positive. Vertical angulations below the occlusal plane are termed as negative. Zero angulations is obtained by kipping PID parallel to the floor

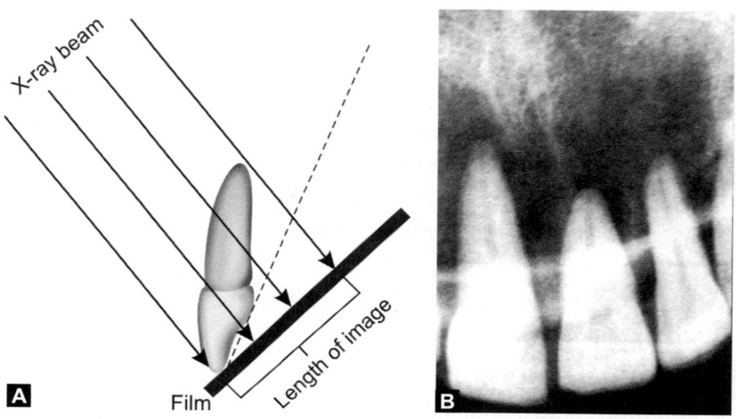

Figs 2.20A and B: A vertical angulation is more than required result in foreshortening of image

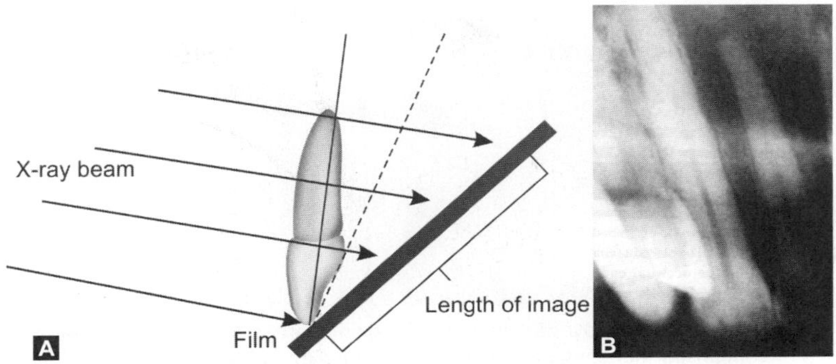

Figs 2.21A and B: A vertical angulations is less than required result in elongation of image

Horizontal Angulation

It is the angulation of the tube in horizontal plane that is side-to-side movement

- In the horizontal plane central ray should be aimed through the interproximal contact areas to avoid overlapping of the teeth
- The horizontal angulation are determined by the shape the arch and position of the teeth
- Incorrect horizontal angulation results in overlapping in the proximal contact area (Fig. 2.22).

Surface Landmark Used for Tube Head Positioning in Bisecting Angle Technique

Maxillary Projection (Table 2.1)

- Horizontal plane—Ala-tragus line is used as reference line and all the point of entry should fall on this plane only
- Vertical plane this differs from teeth to teeth. X-ray cone should be positioned at a point where both the vertical and Horizontal planes meet each other for respective tooth (Figs 2.23 and 2.24).

Incisor: The tube head should be positioned such that the point of entry is through the tip of nose.

Premolar: Point of entry through a point formed by intersection of midpupillary line with the ala-tragus line.

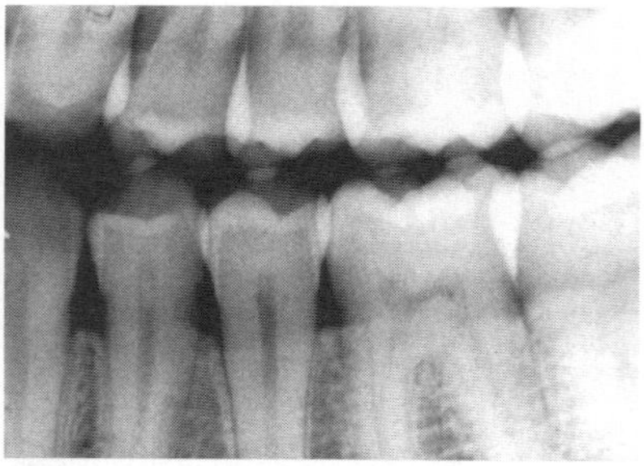

Fig. 2.22: Horizontal overlapping of interproximal areas of crowns is result of improper horizontal angulations (misdirection of the central ray)

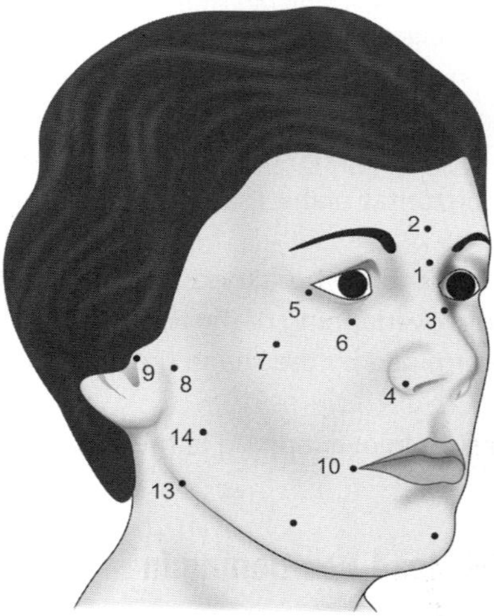

Fig. 2.23: Surface landmarks used for intraoral radiography; 1. Nasion, 2. Glabella, 3. Bridge of nose, 4. Ala of nose, 5. Outer canthus of the eye, 6. Midpoint of infraorbital margin, 7. Zygomatic bone, 8. TMJ articulation, 9. Tragus of the ear, 10. Corner of the mouth, 11. Mid-symphysis, 12. Body of the mandible, 13. Angle of the mandible, 14. Ramus of the mandible

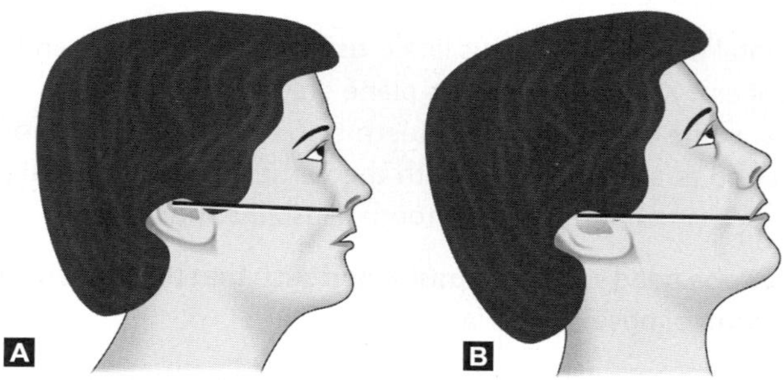

Figs 2.24A and B: Head position for (A) Maxillary teeth; (B) Mandibular teeth

Molar: Central beam is directed through the point of intersection of a line through the outer canthus of eye with ala-tragus line.

Mandibular Projection (Table 2.2)

Horizontal plane center of X-ray cone should be 1 cm above the lower border of mandible.

Vertical plane— It is same as that of maxillary projection.

Advantages of Bisecting Line Angle Technique

- Positioning of the film packet is comfortable for the patient in all areas of the mouth
- It can be used without a film holder
- It can be adapted according to the shape of most dental arch
- Less exposure time is required as short (8 inches PID) is used
- It can be easily undertaken in uncooperative patient as less exposure time is required
- If all angulations are assessed correctly, the image of the tooth will be of the same length as that of the tooth itself and of adequate diagnostic purpose.

Disadvantages of Bisecting Line Angle Technique

- Image distortion: Incorrect vertical angulation, i.e. elongation due to less and foreshortening of image because of increase vertical angulation. Incorrect horizontal angulations can result in overlapping of the proximal surfaces of adjacent teeth
- Required more skill person as horizontal and vertical angles have to be assessed for every patient
- Patients hand is exposed unnecessary to primary beam
- Image cannot be reproduced. As film is hold by patients and vertical angulation and horizontal angulation, i.e. assessed for every exposure
- The periodontal bone level are poorly represented
- The shadow of the zygomatic bone frequently overlies the root of the upper molars
- The crown of the teeth are often distorted, thus preventing the detection of early proximal caries

TABLE 2.1: Details of maxillary radiographs taken by parallel technique

The tooth to be radiographed	Point of entry	Vertical angulation	Exposure parameters	Patients position
Maxillary central incisor	Direct the central ray high on the lip, in the midline, just below the septum of the nostril	+ 40°	65 kVp, 10 mA, 1 second	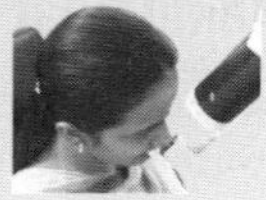
Maxillary lateral incisor	Orient the central ray to enter high on the lip about 1 cm from the midline	+ 40° to + 45°	65 kVp, 10 mA, 1 second	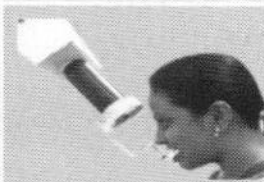
Maxillary canine	Direct the central ray through the canine eminence. The point of entry will be about the intersection of the distal and inferior borders of the ala of the nose	+ 45°	65 kVp, 10 mA, 1 second	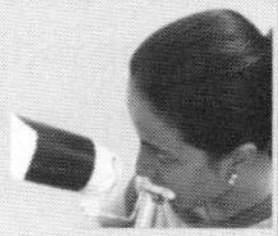
Maxillary premolars	Central ray should pass through the center of the second premolar root; the point of entry usually is below the pupil of the eye	+ 30°	65 kVp, 10 mA, $1^{1/4}$ second	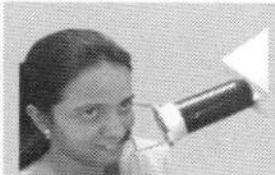
Maxillary molars	The point of entry should be on the cheek below the outer canthus of the eye and the zygoma at the position of the maxillary second molar	+ 20°	65 kVp, 0 mA, $1^{1/2}$ second	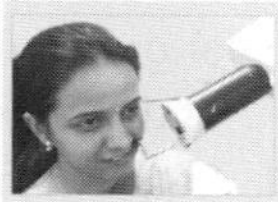
Maxillary distal oblique molar	The central ray enters the maxillary third molar region just below the middle of the zygomatic arch, distal to the lateral canthus of the eye	+ 20°	65kVp, 10 mA, $1^{1/2}$ second	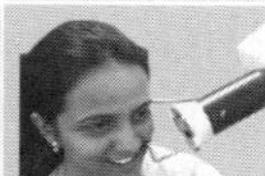

TABLE 2.2: Details of mandibular radiographs taken by bisecting angle technique

The tooth to be radiographed	Point of entry	Vertical angulation	Exposure parameters	Patients position
Mandibular central and lateral incisor	The central ray is directed below the lower lip and about 1 cm lateral to the midline	– 15	65 kVp, 10 mA, 1 second	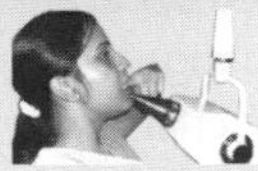
Mandibular canine	The point of entry is nearly perpendicular to the ala of the nose, over the position of the canine, and about 3 cm above the inferior border of the mandible	– 20	65 kVp, 10 mA, $1^{1/2}$ second	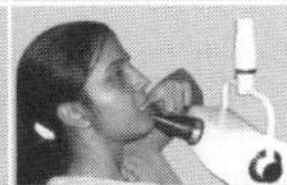
Mandibular premolar	The central ray is oriented below the pupil of the eye and about 3 cm above the inferior border of the mandible	– 10	65 kVp, 10 mA, $1^{1/4}$ second	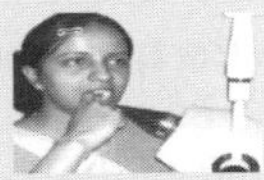
Mandibular molar	The point of entry is below the outer canthus of the eye about 3 cm above the inferior border of the mandible	– 5	65 kVp, 10 mA, $1^{1/2}$ second	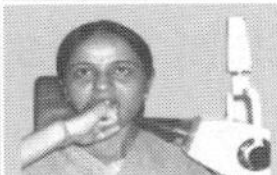
Mandibular distal oblique molar	Orient the point of entry about 3 cm above the antegonial notch on the inferior border of the mandible, in line with the anterior border of the ramus	– 5	65 kVp, 10 mA, $1^{1/2}$ second	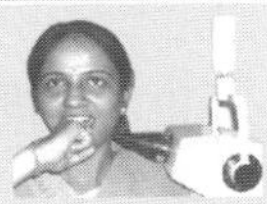

INTRAORAL LOCALIZATION TECHNIQUES

There are two basic methods for object localization in the jaw. These methods used to locate the position of the tooth or an object in the jaw. Foreign bodies, impacted teeth, retained roots salivary stones, jaw fractures, broken needles and instrument root position.

Tube Shift Technique or Clerks Rule (Buccal Object Rules)

The basic principal is that relative position of the radiographic image of two separate objects changes, when the projection angle (horizontal) is changed. To locate the vertically aligned image horizontal angle should be changed, and to locate the horizontal aligned images the vertical angle should be changed.

Two radiograph of the same object are taken. First using the proper technique and angulations.

And second radiograph is taken keeping all others parameter constant only changing the direction of central beam with different horizontal or vertical angulation.

Interpretation: When the object seen in the second radiograph appears to have moved in the same direction as the shift of central beam, the object in the question is said to be positioned lingually (Figs 2.25A and B).

But if the object appears to have moved in a direction opposite to the slnift central ray, then the object is question is said to be positioned buccaly. SLOB: Same lingual, opposite buccal.

Right Angle Technique

Two projections are taken at right angles to each other, which helps to localize an object in the maxilla or mandible.

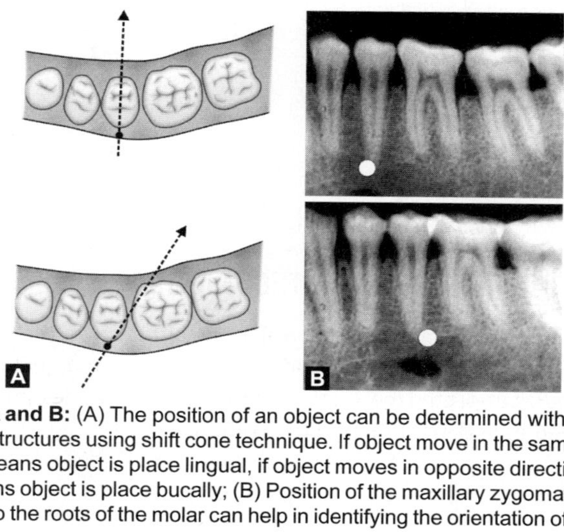

Figs 2.25A and B: (A) The position of an object can be determined with respect to reference structures using shift cone technique. If object move in the same direction of tube it means object is place lingual, if object moves in opposite direction to cone shift it means object is place bucally; (B) Position of the maxillary zygomatic process in relation to the roots of the molar can help in identifying the orientation of projection

A periapical radiograph is taken to show the position of the object superior inferiorly anterior posterior. Occlusal radiograph is taken which will show the object bucco-lingual and anteroposterior relationship. There two radiographs when studied together help to localize the object in all three dimensions (Figs 2.26 and 2.27).

EXTRAORAL RADIOGRAPHY

Extraoral radiography utilizes the screen film in cassettes equipped with screens. Screen-film combination is faster than the film alone and therefore, one can make the radiograph with reasonably short exposure time and thus reduces the radiation to the patient. Usually the cassettes come in different sizes such as 5 × 7", 8 × 10", 10 × 12" and 5 × 12". There are two types of screens used with these cassettes. They are made up of either

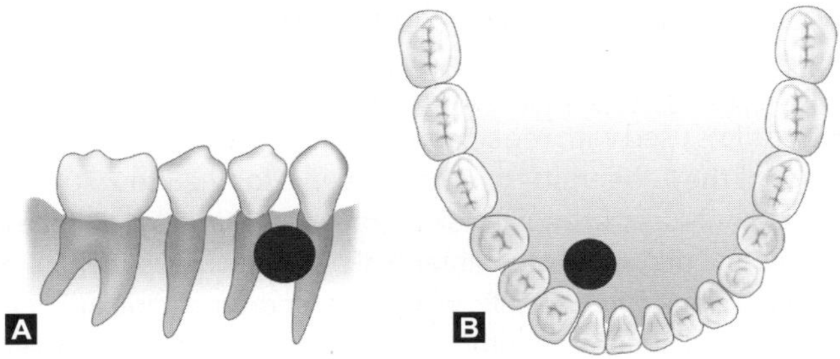

Figs 2.26A and B: (A) In periapical radiograph, object appears to be in bone; (B) Occlusal radiograph shows that the object is actually located in the soft tissue lingual to the mandible

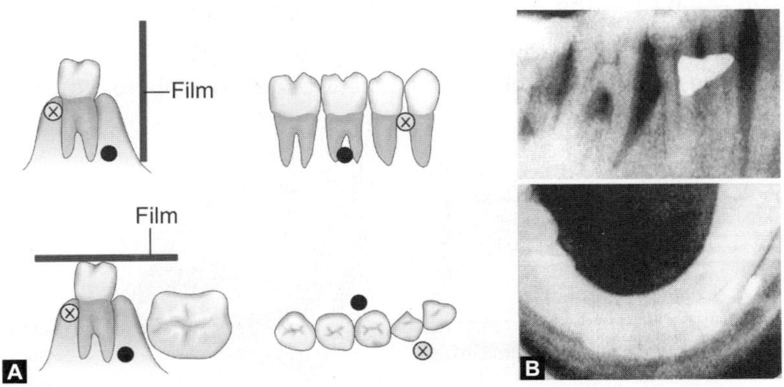

Figs 2.27A and B: Two films are exposed at right angle to each other to identify the location of an object (Periapical and occlusal view)

calcium tungstate or rare earth material. The calcium tungstate screen gives out a blue light, while rare earth screen gives out a green light when exposed to X-rays.

Indication for Extraoral Radiograph

- Patients having trismus
- To examine the extent of lesions
- Examination of large area of jaw bone
- To evaluate trauma
- To evaluate impacted teeth
- To evaluate temporomandibular joint.

An important aspect of the extraoral radiography technique is the immobilization of patients. These radiographs are useful in cases of trauma, trismus or any other reason due to which the patient is unable to open the mouth.

Extraoral radiography utilizes the screen film in cassettes equipped with screens. The films used with the screen are made to be specifically sensitive to the color of the light emitted by the screen (Figs 2.28 to 2.30).

The commonly used extraoral radiographs include a lateral oblique view of the mandible and maxilla, posteroanterior (PA) view of mandible, lateral skull, PA skull, lateral sinus, three specific view for temporomandibular joint (TMJ), Towne's projection, Bregma mentum view and submentovertex projection.

Surface landmarks used in extraoral radiography for patient positioning: (Figs 2.31A and B).

The Median Plane of the Head (Midsagittal Plane)

This is determined by a line that is coincident with the sagittal suture between the upper margins of the parietal bones, running from the top of the skull backward.

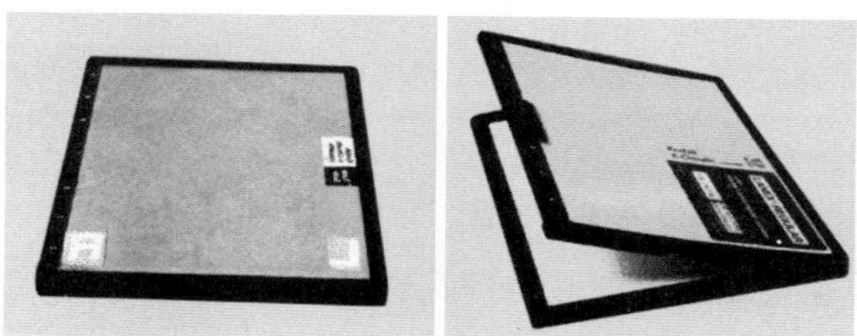

Fig. 2.28: Extraoral cassette 8 × 10 inch and partially open cassette

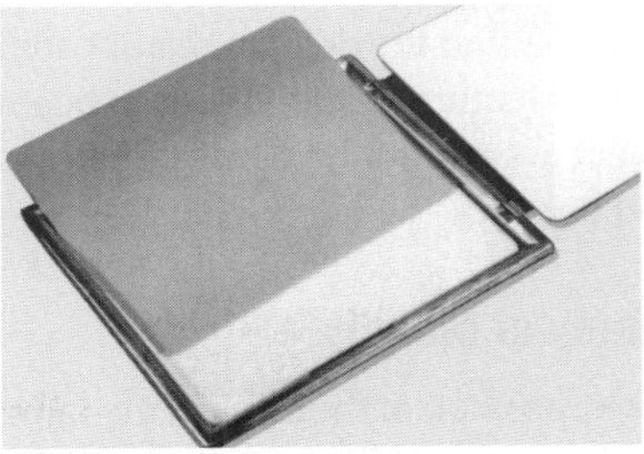

Fig. 2.29: Extraoral cassette in open position showing intensifying screens

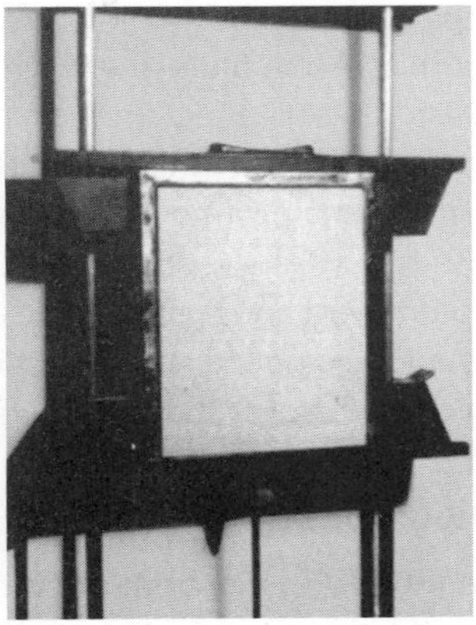

Fig. 2.30: Extraoral cassette in wall mounted film holding device

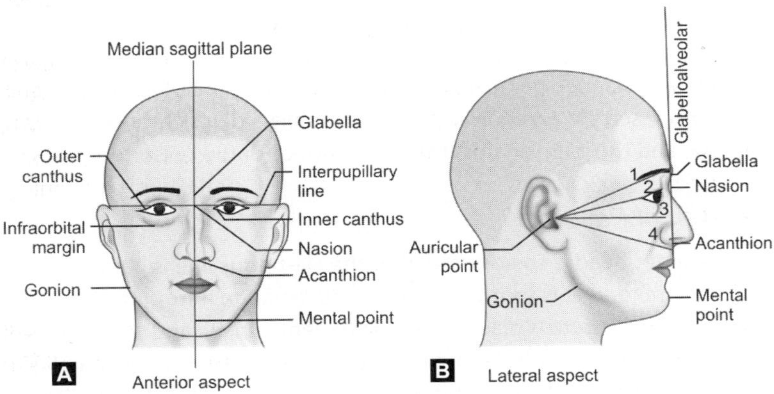

Figs 2.31A and B: External guide lines used for patients' position in anterior aspect and in lateral aspect

For lateral views the median plane is kept parallel with the cassette. And for posteroanterior and anteroposterior views, the median plane is kept at right angles to the film cassettes.

The film focus distance importance is paramount. An increase in the focus film distance will improve the image sharpness, but adequate collimation must be used to prevent scattered radiation. Longer the film focus distance, the image is produced by more of the central rays, which in turn give minimum alteration in the true anatomical size. The film focus distance has no effect on the radiographic contrast obtained.

Most of the techniques for skull radiography use a film focus distance of approximately three feet (90 cm), in cephalometry a distance of 5–6 feet (150–180 cm) are used. It is useful to bear in mind the definite relationship to prominent and recognizable anatomical features and the central beam should be so directed as to pass or project away from the dense structures which would over shadow the required details.

Lateral Oblique View (Anterior Body of Mandible)

Image field: Anterior body of the mandible, position of the teeth in the same area. It helps to evaluate impacted teeth, fractures and lesions located in the inferior border of the mandible.

Position of Film

The cassette is placed flat against the patient's cheek and is centered over the body of the mandible, overlying the canine teeth. The cassette also should be positioned parallel to the body of the mandible. The patient must hold the cassette in position with the thumb placed under the edge of the cassette and the palm against the outer surface of the cassette.

Position of Patients

The patient's head is so adjusted, that the ala-tragus line is parallel to the floor. The mandible is protruded slightly to separate it from the vertebral column. The cassette is placed over the patient's cheek and centered over the area of interest. The inferior border of the cassette should be parallel to the lower border of the mandible and below it. The sagittal plane is tilted so that it is 5° to the vertical, and rotated 30° from the true lateral position. For the bicuspid and incisor region, the patient's head can be turned slightly away from the tube so that the nose and chin approximate the cassette.

Direction of central beam: Is directed from under the mandible opposite to the side of examination, from 2 cm behind the angle of the mandible. The beam is directed upward (–10° to –15°) and centered on the anterior body of the mandible. The beam must be directed perpendicular to the horizontal plane of the film (Fig. 2.32).

Exposure parameter: kVp- 65-70, mA-7-10, seconds-0.8

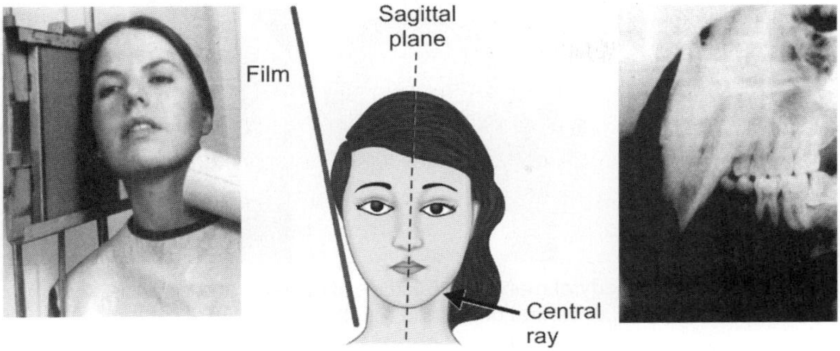

Fig. 2.32: Lateral oblique projection: Position of patients and cassette, direction of central beam and resultant image

Posterior Body of the Mandible

Image Field

Body of the mandible, position of the teeth in the same area, ramus of the mandible, angle of the mandible. It helps to evaluate impacted teeth, fractures and lesions located in the inferior border of the mandible.

Position of Film

The cassette is placed flat against the patient's cheek and is centered over the body of the mandible. The cassette also should be positioned parallel to the body of the mandible. The patient must hold the cassette in position with the thumb placed under the edge of the cassette and the palm against the outer surface of the cassette.

Position of Patients

The patient's head is so adjusted, that the ala-tragus line is parallel to the floor. The mandible is protruded slightly to separate it from the vertebral column. The cassette is placed over the patient's cheek and centered over the area of interest.

The inferior border of the cassette should be parallel to the lower border of the mandible and below it. The sagittal plane is tilted so that it is 50° to the vertical and the head is rotated 10°–15° from the true lateral position.

For the molar and ramus region, the head should not be turned away from the tube as this will place the ramus behind the vertebral column.

Direction of central beam: Is directed from under the mandible opposite the side of examination, from 2 cm below the angle of the mandible. The beam is directed upward (–10° to –15°) and centered on the body of the mandible. The beam must be directed perpendicular to the horizontal plane of the film (Fig. 2.33).

Exposure parameter: kVp-65-70, mA-7-10, 0.8 seconds

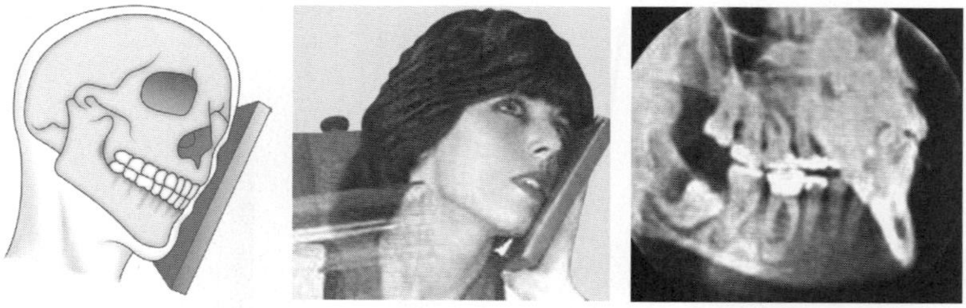

Fig. 2.33: Posterior body of mandible: Position of patients and cassette, direction of central beam and resultant image

Ramus of Mandible

Image Field

The purpose of this view is to evaluate impacted third molars, large lesions, fractures that extend into the ramus of the mandible. This projection demonstrates a view of the ramus from the angle of the mandible to the condyles.

Film Position

The cassette is placed flat against the patient's cheek and is centered over the ramus of the mandible. The cassette also should be positioned parallel to the ramus of the mandible. The patient must hold the cassette in position with the thumb placed under the edge of the cassette and the palm against the outer surface of the cassette.

Position of Patients

The patient's head is so adjusted, that the ala-tragus line is parallel to the floor. The mandible is protruded slightly to separate it from the vertebral column. The cassette is placed over the patient's cheek and centered over the area of interest.

The inferior border of the cassette should be parallel to the lower border of the mandible and below it. The sagittal plane is tilted so that it is 10° to the vertical and the head is rotated 5° from the true lateral position.

Direction of central beam: Is directed from under the mandible opposite the side of examination, from behind the angle of the mandible to a point posterior to the third molar region on the side opposite the cassette. The beam is directed upward (–10° to –15°) and centered on the ramus of the mandible. The beam must be directed perpendicular to the horizontal plane of the film (Fig. 2.34).

Exposure parameter: kVp-65-70, mA-7-10, 0.8 seconds

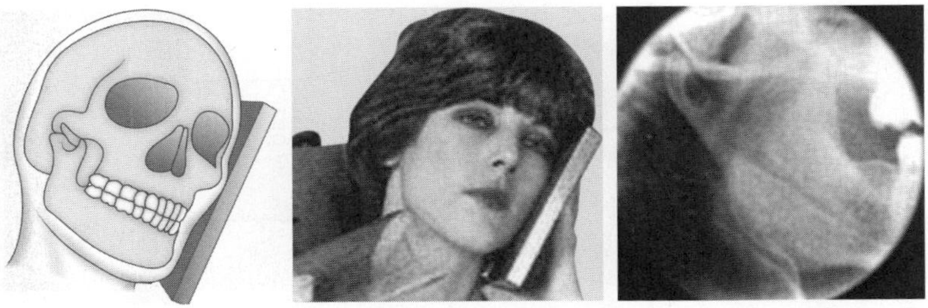

Fig. 2.34: Ramus of mandible: Position of patients and cassette, direction of central beam and resultant image

POSTEROANTERIOR PROJECTION (ALSO KNOWN AS THE OCCIPITOFRONTAL PROJECTION OF THE NASAL SINUSES)

There are two methods for obtaining this projection:

A. Posteroanterior (Granger) projection.
B. Inclined posteroanterior (Caldwell) projection.

Posteroanterior (Granger) Projection

Image Field

This view is excellent for evaluating the inner and middle ear because the petrous pyramid can be viewed through the orbits. Frontal sinuses lying above the frontonasal suture, anterior ethmoidal cells lying each on either side of the nasal fossa, sphenoidal sinuses projected through the nasal fossa just below or between the shadows of the ethmoids. The upper part of the antrum is superimposed by dense shadows of the petrosae.

Position of Film

The cassette is placed perpendicular to the floor in a cassette holding device. The long axis of the cassette is positioned vertically.

Position of Patients

The midsagittal plane should be vertical and perpendicular to the plane of the cassette. Only the forehead and nose should touch the cassette. The radiographic baseline is at 90° to the film.

Direction of central beam: Is directed to the midline of the skull so that the X-ray beam passes through the canthomeatal plane perpendicular to the film plane (Figs 2.35 and 2.36).

Exposure parameter: kVp-65, mA-10, 3 seconds

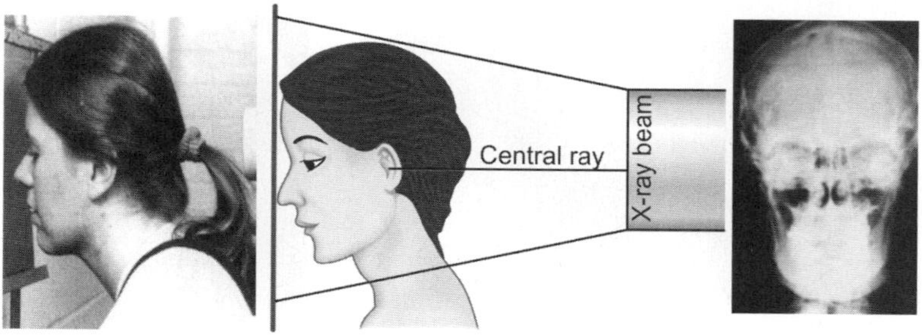

Fig. 2.35: Posterioanterior view: Position of patients and cassette, direction of central beam and resultant image

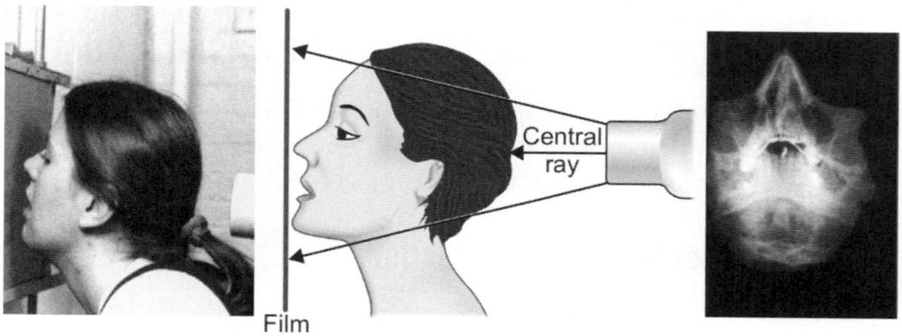

Fig. 2.36: Waters view: Position of patients and cassette, direction of central beam and resultant image

Inclined Posteroanterior (Caldwell) Projection

Image Field

This angulation will cause the petrous ridges to be superimposed on the maxillary sinuses, thus allowing more accurate examination of the orbits and ethmoidal air cells.

Position of Film

The cassette is placed perpendicular to the floor in a cassette holding device. The long-axis of the cassette is positioned vertically.

Position of Patients

The midsagittal plane is vertical and perpendicular to the cassette. Only the forehead and nose touch the cassette, so that the canthomeatalline is perpendicular to the cassette. On the resultant radiograph the superior border of the petrous ridge is projected in the lower third of the orbit.

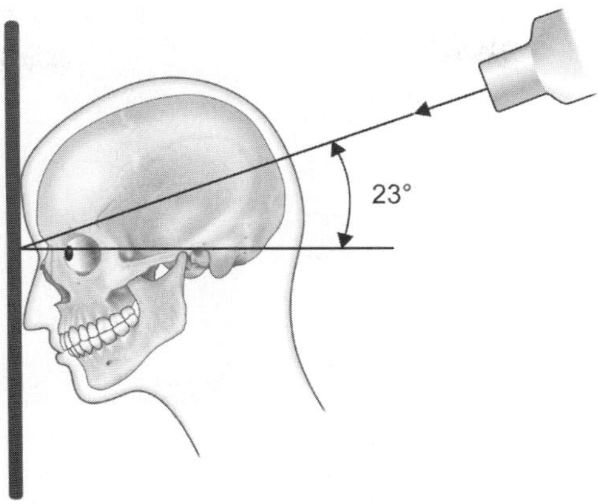

Figs 2.37: Caldwell projection: Position of patients and cassette, direction of central beam

Direction of Central Beam

It is directed 23° to the canthomeatalline, entering the skull about 3 cm above the external occipital protuberance and exiting at the glabella (Fig. 2.37)

Exposure parameter: kVp-65, mA-10, 3 seconds

RADIOGRAPHY OF THE MAXILLARY SINUSES

Standard Occipitomental Projection (0° OM)

Image Field

The projection shows the facial skeleton and the maxillary antra, and avoids superimposition of the dense bones of the base of the skull. It is especially useful to detect middle third fracture (LeFort I,II,III, zygomatic complex, nasoethmoidal complex, orbital blowout) and coronoid fractures.

Position of Film

The cassette is placed perpendicular to the floor in a cassette holding device. The long-axis of the cassette is positioned vertically.

Position of Patients

The midsagittal plane should be vertical and perpendicular to the plane of the cassette. Only the nose and chin should touch the cassette. The head is tipped back so that the radiographic baseline is at 45° to the film.

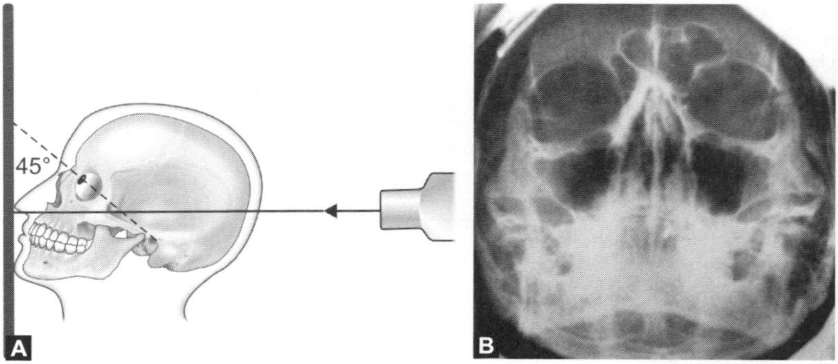

Figs 2.38A and B: Standard occipitomental projection (0°): Position of patients and cassette, direction of central beam and resultant image

Direction of Central Beam

Is directed horizontally through the occiput (Figs 2.38A and B)

Exposure parameter: kVp-6,. mA-10, 2–3 seconds

Modified Method (30° Occipitomental Projection)

Image Field

This projection shows the facial skeleton, from a different angle enabling certain bony displacements to be detected. It is useful in detecting middle third fractures (LeFort I, II and III) and coronoid process fractures.

Position of Film

The cassette is placed perpendicular to the floor in a cassette holding device. The long axis of the cassette is positioned vertically.

Position of Patients

The midsagittal plane is vertical and perpendicular to the cassette. The head is centered so that the nasion is in the center of the cassette.

Only the nose and chin touch the cassette, the head is tipped back so that the radiographic baseline is at 45° to the film.

Direction of Central Beam

Is directed 30° to the horizontal, centered through the lower border of the orbit (Figs 2.39A and B).

Exposure parameter: kVp-65, mA-10, 2–3 seconds

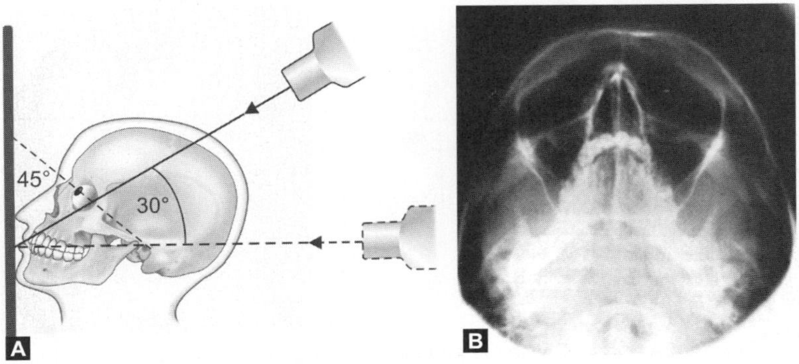

Figs 2.39A and B: Modified occipitomental projection (30°): Position of patients and cassette, direction of central beam and resultant image

Posteroanterior Water's

Image Field

This projection is primarily used to demonstrate the maxillary sinus, frontal and ethmoidal sinuses.

The sphenoidal sinuses can be seen if the patient is asked to open his mouth, whereby the sphenoidal sinuses are projected on the palate.

The orbit, frontozygomatic suture, nasal cavity, coronoid process of the mandible and the zygomatic arch are also seen.

Film Position

The cassette is placed perpendicular to the floor in a cassette holding device. The long-axis of the cassette is positioned vertically.

Patients Position

The midsagittal plane should be vertical and perpendicular to the plane of the film. The patient's head is extended so that only the chin touches the cassette.

The cassette is centered around the acanthion (anterior nasal spine). The canthomeatalline should be at 37° to the plane of the film and the line from the external auditory meatus to the mental protuberance should be perpendicular to the film.

Water's (1915) specified that the tip of the nose should be 0.5–1.5 cm away from the cassette; Mahoney (1930) found that the petrosal shadows can be correctly placed by adjusting the orbitomeatalline at 37° to the horizontal.

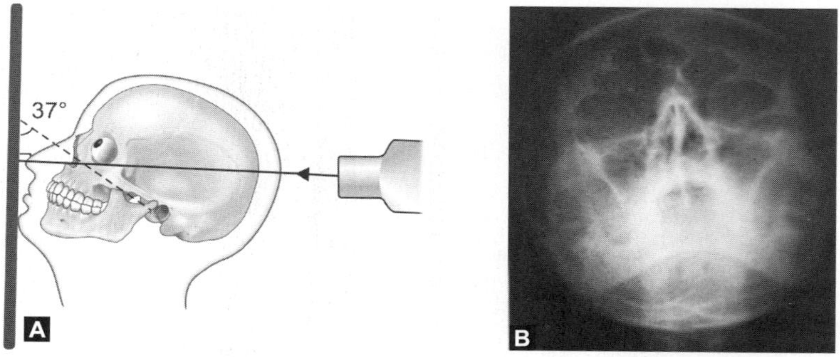

Figs 2.40A and B: PA waters projection: Position of patients and cassette, direction of central beam and resultant image

Direction of Central Beam

It is directed perpendicular and to the midpoint of the film. It enters from the vertex and exists from the acanthion (Figs 2.40A and B)

Exposure parameter: kVp-65, mA-10, 2–3 seconds.

Bregma Menton

Image Field

This projection is primarily used to demonstrate the walls of the maxillary sinus (especially in the posterior areas), the orbits, the zygomatic arches and the nasal septum. It also demonstrates medial or lateral deviations of any part of the mandible.

Film Position

The cassette is placed perpendicular to the floor in a cassette holding device. The long-axis of the cassette is positioned vertically.

Position of Patients

The midsagittal plane should be vertical and perpendicular to the plane of the film.The patient's head is extended as far as comfortable, to make the lower border of the mandible as parallel to the cassette as possible. Only the chin touches the cassette. The canthomeatal line should also be approximately parallel to the plane of the film.

Direction of Central Beam

The central ray enters at the bregma and exits at the menton (Figs 2.41A and B).

Exposure parameter: kVp-65, mA-10, 2–3 seconds

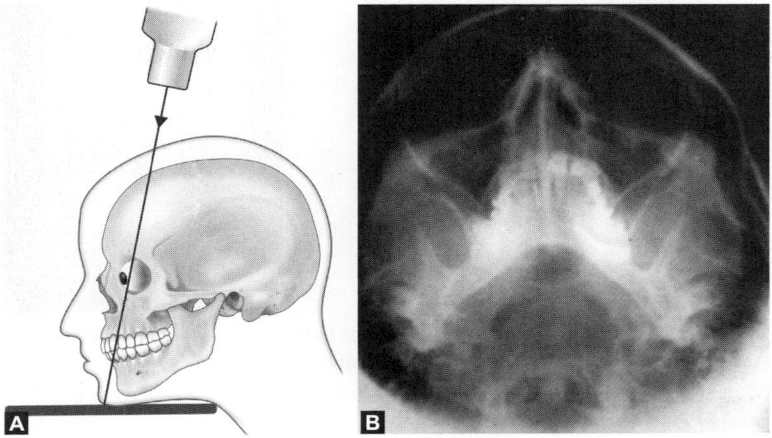

Figs 2.41A and B: Bregma menton view: Position of patients and cassette, direction of central beam and resultant image

RADIOGRAPHY OF THE MANDIBLE

Posteroanterior Mandible

Image Field

A posteroanterior (PA) projection of the mandibular body and the ramus. The central part of the body is not well seen because of the superimposition of the spine. It is used to study fractures of the posterior third of the body of the mandible, angles, rami and lower condylar necks, mediolateral expansion of the posterior third of the body or the rami in case of tumors or cystic lesions, maxillofacial deformities and mandibular hypoplasia or hyperplasia.

Position of Film

The cassette is placed perpendicular to the floor in a cassette holding device. The long-axis of the cassette is positioned vertically.

Position of Patients

The sagittal plane should be vertical and perpendicular to the film. The head is tipped downward so that the forehead and nose touch the film. The radiographic base line is horizontal and perpendicular to the film. The film is adjusted so that the lips are centered to the film.

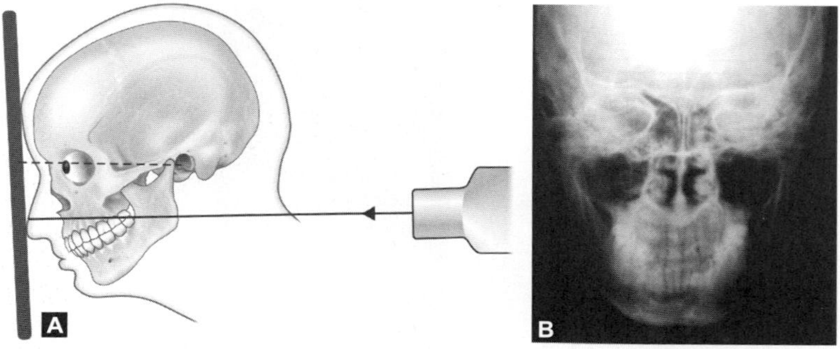

Figs 2.42A and B: PA mandible: Position of patients and cassette, direction of central beam and resultant image

Direction of Central Beam

It is directed at right angles to the film through the midsagittal plane through the cervical spine, at the level of the angles of the mandible (Figs 2.42A and B).

Exposure parameter: kVp-65, mA-10, 2–3 seconds.

Rotated PA Mandible

Image Field

This projection is used to show the tissues of one side of the face and used to investigate the parotid gland and the ramus of the mandible. It is mainly used to demonstrate, stones or calculi in the parotid, to note the mediolateral expansion of lesions in the ramus and submasseteric infections.

Film Position

The cassette is placed perpendicular to the floor in a cassette holding device. The long-axis of the cassette is positioned vertically.

Position of Patients

The patient is positioned facing the film, with the occlusal plane horizontal and the tip of the nose touching the film.The head is rotated 10° to the side of interest. This rotates the bones of the back of the skull away from the side of the face.

Direction of Central Beam

It is directed at right angles to the film, aimed down the side (Figs 2.43A to C).

Exposure parameter: kVp-65. mA-7, 2 seconds

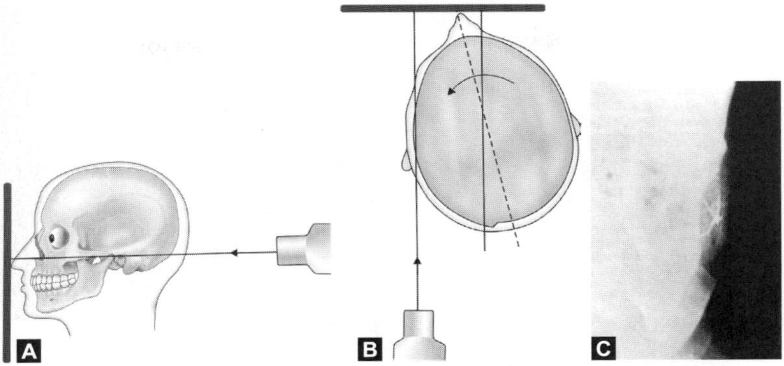

Figs 2.43A to C: Rotated PA mandible: Position of patients and cassette, direction of central beam and resultant image

RADIOGRAPHY OF TEMPOROMANDIBULAR JOINT

Transcranial View

Image Field

Technique is most useful in detecting arthritic changes he articular surface. It helps to evaluate the joint's bony relationship. It changes on the central and medial surfaces are not seen.

Position of Film

The cassette is placed flat against the patient's ear and covered over the temporomadibular joint (TMJ) of interest, against the facial parallel to the sagittal plane.

Position of Patients

Patients head is adjusted in such a way that the sagittal plane is vertical. The ala tragus line is parallel to floor. This view is taken in close and open mouth position.

Direction of Central Beam

Central ray enters through a point 2″ above the external auditory meatus. or ½″ behind and 2″ above the external auditory meatus or ½″ anterior and 2″ above the external auditory meatus. In all the three type the central ray is directed caudally at the angle of 20°–25°. The point of exit is through the of interest (Figs 2.44A to C).

Exposure parameter: kVp-70, mA-7, 1.5 seconds

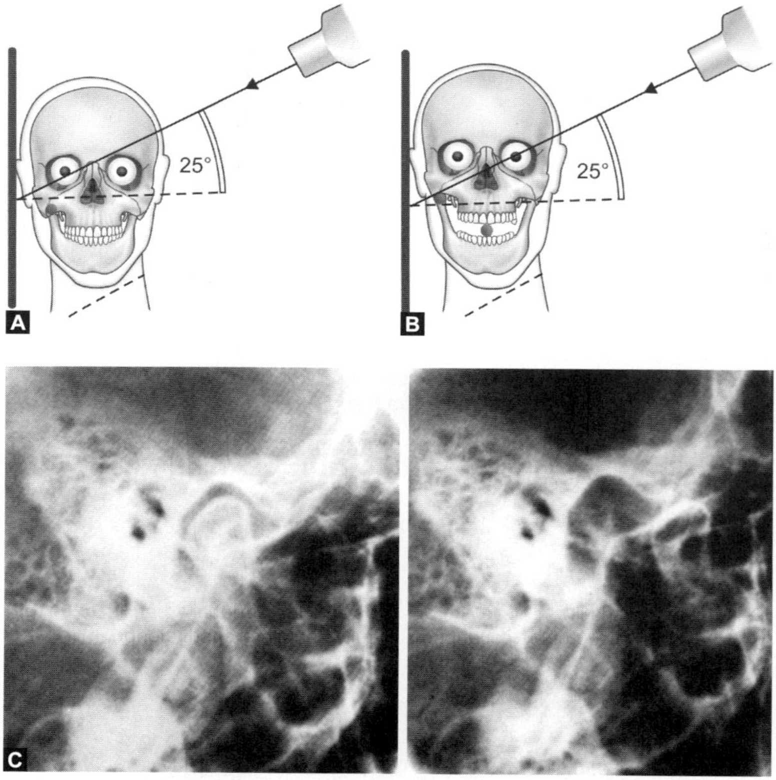

Figs 2.44A to C: Transcranial view: Position of patients and cassette, direction of central beam and resultant image of closed and open mouth position

Transpharyngeal (Infracranial or McQueen Dell Technique)

Image Field

This view is a lateral projection of the condylar head and neck, usually taken in the mouth open position, so that the joint is projected into the shadow of air containing spaces of the nasopharynx, which helps to increase the contrast of the various parts of the joint.

Position of Film

The cassette is placed flat against the patient's ear and is centered to a point Yz" anterior to the external auditory meatus, over the TMJ of interest, against the facial skin parallel to the sagittal plane.

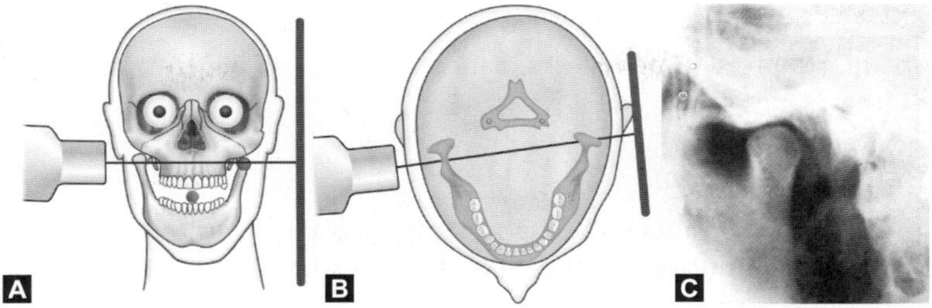

Figs 2.45A to C: Transpharyngeal view: (A) Position of patients and cassette; (B) Direction of central beam; (C) Resultant image (Open mouth position)

Position of Patients

The patient is positioned so that the sagittal plane is vertical and parallel to the film, with the TMJ of interest adjacent to the film.

The film is centered to a point Yz" anterior to the external auditory meatus.

The occlusal plane should be parallel to the transverse axis of the film so that the soft parts of the nasopharynx are in one line with the TMJ. The patient is instructed to slowly inhale through the nose during exposure, so as to ensure filling of the nasopharynx with air during the exposure. The patient should open his mouth so that the condyles move away from the base of the skull and the mandibular notch of the opposite side is enlarged.

Direction of Central Beam

It is directed from the opposite side cranially, at an angle of –5° to –10° posteriorly. It is directed through the mandibular notch, which is a window between the coronoid, condyle and the zygomatic arch, of the side below the base of the skull to the TMJ of interest (Figs 2.45A to C).

Exposure parameter: kVp-70. mA-7, 0.8 seconds

Transorbital (Zimmer Projection)

It is the conventional frontal TMJ projection which is most successful in delineating the joint with minimal super impositions, leading to the production of a relatively true enface' projection.

Image Field

The anterior view of the TM joint and medial displacement of fractured condyle and fracture of condyle are seen in this view.

Position of Film

The film is position behind the patients head at an angle of 45° to the sagittal plane.

Position of Patients

The patients is positioned so that the sagittal plane is vertical.

The canthomeatal line should be 10° to the horizontal, with the head tipped downward with wide open mouth.

Direction of Central Beam

The tube head is placed in front of the patient's face. The central ray is directed to the joint of interest, at an angle of +20°, to strike the cassette at right angles (Figs 2.46A to C).

The point of entry may be taken at:

- ❑ Pupil of the same eye, asking the patient to look straight ahead
- ❑ Medial canthus of the same eye
- ❑ Medial canthus of the opposite eye.

Using Intraoral X-ray Machine

Exposure parameter: kVp-70, mA-7-10, 0.8 seconds

Using Extraoral X-ray Machine

Exposure parameter: kVp-40, mA-40, 1 second

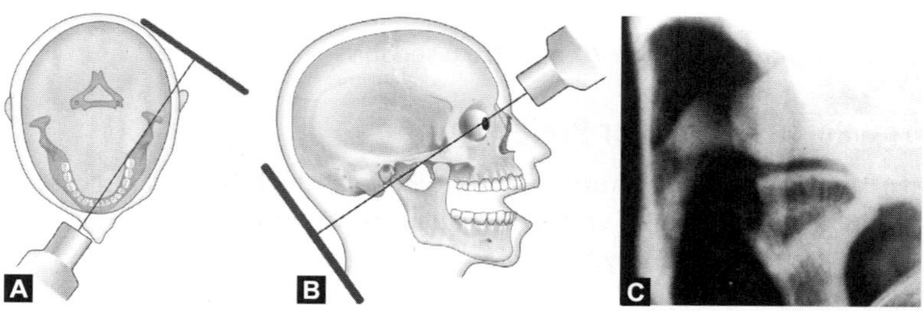

Figs 2.46A to C: Transorbital view: Position of patients and cassette, direction of central beam and resultant image

RADIOGRAPHY OF THE BASE OF THE SKULL

Submentovertex Projection

Image Field

A full axial view of the base of the cranium showing a symmetrical projection of the petrosa, the mastoid process, foramen ovale, spinosum canals, carotid canals, sphenoidal sinuses, mandible, maxillary sinus, nasal septum, odontoid process of the atlas and the entire atlas, axial inclination of the mandibular condyles. It helps to study destructive/expansile lesions affecting the palate, pterygoid region or base of the skull, sphenoidal sinus.

Position of Film

The cassette is placed perpendicular to the floor in a cassette holding device. The long-axis of the cassette is placed horizontally.

Position of Patients

The head is centered on the cassette, with the patient's head and neck tipped back as far as possible, the vertex (top) of the skull touches the cassette. Both the midsagittal plane should be perpendicular to the plane of the film and the radiographic base line should be parallel to the film.

Direction of Central Beam

It is directed perpendicular to the film. It enters through the midsagittal plane, between the angles of the mandible and in a coronal plane 3/4th inches anterior to the external auditory meatus.

In order to view the petrous portion, the central ray is directed at right angles (or 5° to the horizontal) to the film midway between the external auditory meatus (Figs 2.47A to C).

Exposure parameter: kVp-65, mA- 20–30, OA seconds

RADIOGRAPHY OF THE ZYGOMATIC ARCHES

Jug Handle View (A Modification of the Submentovertex View)

Image Field

A symmetrical axial view of the zygomatic arches.

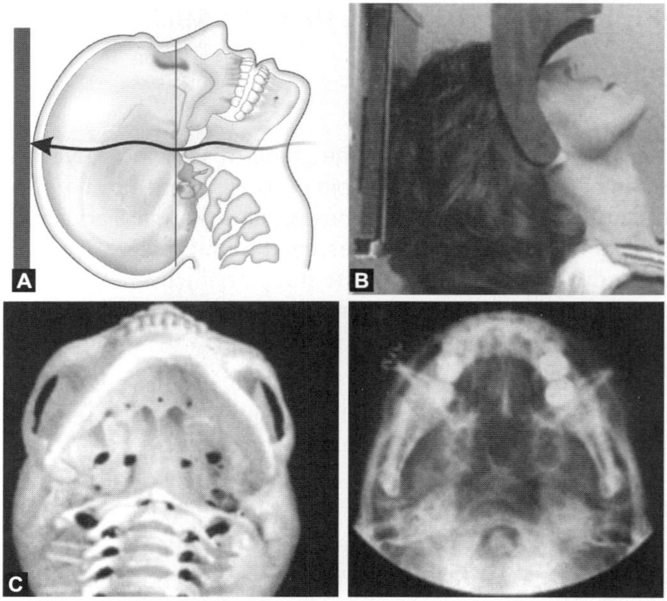

Figs 2.47A to C: Submentovertex projection: Position of patients and cassette, direction of central beam and resultant image

Position of Film

The cassette is placed perpendicular to the floor in a cassette holding device. The long-axis of the cassette is placed horizontally.

Position of Patients

The head is centered on the cassette, with the patient's head and neck tipped back as far as possible, the vertex (top) of the skull touches the cassette. Both the midsagittal plane should be perpendicular to the plane of the film and the radiographic base line should be parallel to the film.

Direction of Central Beam

The cone is brought as close as possible to the patient, which leads to magnification of the structures at the base of the skull (Fig. 2.48).

Exposure parameter: kVp-65. mA-20–30, OA seconds. The exposure time for the zygomatic arch is reduced to approximately one-third of the normal exposure time for a submentovertex projection.

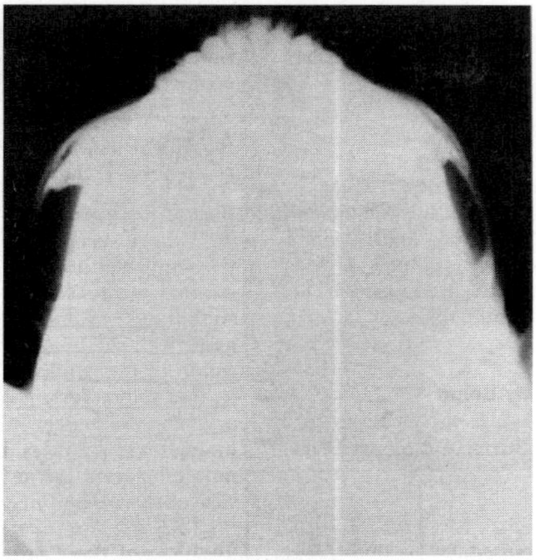

Fig. 2.48: Modified submentovertex projection (Jug-Handle view): Position of patients and cassette, direction of central beam and resultant image

Reverse Townes

Image Field

This view is primarily meant for viewing the condylar neck and head. High fractures of the condylar necks, intra capsular fractures of the TMJ, quality of articular surfaces, condylar hypoplasia or hypertrophy.

Film Position

The cassette is placed perpendicular to the floor in a cassette holding device. The long-axis of the cassette is placed vertically.

Position of Patients

The position of the patient is the same as that in PA mandible, i.e. the sagittal plane should be vertical and perpendicular to the film. The film is adjusted so that the lips are centered to the film.

Only the patient's forehead and tip of the nose should touch the film.

The only difference being that the patient here is asked to keep his/her mouth wide open and the radiographic base line is at an angle of negative 30° to the film.

Direction of Central Beam

It is directed through the midsagittal plane at the level of the mandible, and is perpendicular to the film (Figs 2.49A to C).

Exposure parameter: kVp-65, mA-10, 2–3 seconds

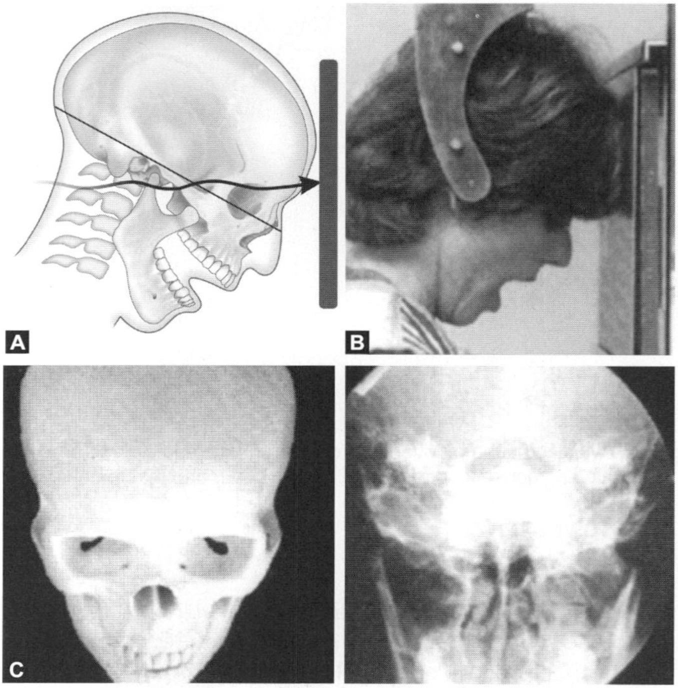

Figs 2.49A to C: Reverse towne's projection: Position of patients and cassette, direction of central beam and resultant image

SKULL PROJECTION

Lateral Cephalogram

Image Field

This view is used to evaluate facial growth and development, trauma, disease and developmental anomalies.

This projection demonstrates the bones of the face, skull as well as the soft tissue profile of the face.

The soft tissue outline of the face is more readily seen on the resulting radiograph when a filter is used. A filter is placed at the X-ray source, or between the patient and the film, and serves to remove some of the X-rays that pass through the soft tissue of the face, thus enhancing the image of the soft tissue profile.

In oral surgery and prosthetics it is used to establish pretreatment and post-treatment records.

Position of Film

The cassette is placed perpendicular to the floor with the long axis of the cassette placed vertically (FFD is the largest, 5 feet).

Position of Patients

The left side of the patient's head is positioned against the cassette. The midsagittal plane is perpendicular to the floor and parallel to the film/cassette.

The patient's head is stabilized with the help of the ear rods, nasion positioner and the orbital rod.

The patient is asked to keep the teeth in occlusion.

Direction of Central Beam

The central ray is directed perpendicular to the cassette through the porion. The distance between the X-ray source and the midcoronal plane of the patient is 60 inches (Figs 2.50A to C).

Exposure parameter: kVp-84. mA-13, 1.6 seconds

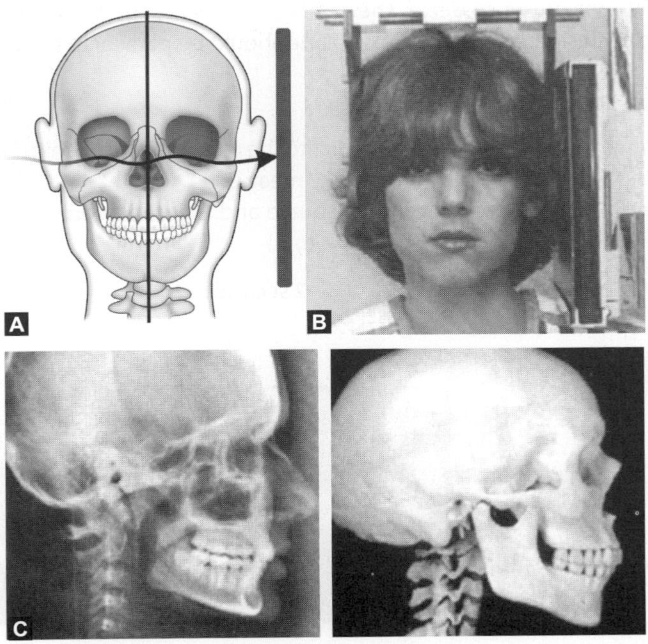

Figs 2.50A to C: Lateral cephalogram: Position of patients and cassette, direction of central beam and resultant image

True Lateral

Image Field

It is used to survey the skull and facial bones for evidence of trauma, disease or developmental abnormality. This view reveals the nasopharyngeal soft tissues, paranasal sinuses and hard palate.

Conditions affecting the sella turcica, such as tumors of the pituitary gland in acromegaly.

Position of Film

The film is held vertically against the patient's cheek and centered so that the entire skull is along with the facial skeleton, is seen on the resultant radiograph.

Position of Patients

The sagittal plane should be vertical and parallel to the film. The film is adjusted so that the upper circumference of the skull is Yz inch below the upper border of the cassette. The patient here is asked to keep his/her teeth in occlusion, and the occlusal plane should be parallel to the floor.

Direction of Central Beam

The central ray is directed perpendicular to the cassette and the midsagittal plane and toward the external auditory meatus.

The distance between the X-ray source and the midcoronal plane of the patient is 36–40 inches (Figs 2.51A to C)

Exposure Parameter: kVp-65. mA-I0, 0.5–2 seconds

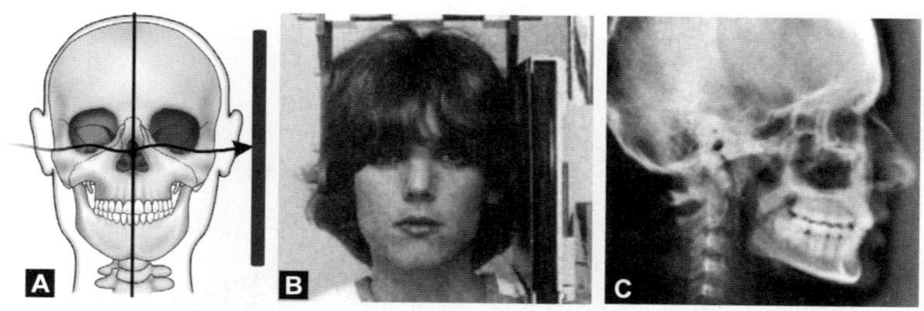

Figs 2.51A to C: True lateral projection: Position of patients and cassette, direction of central beam and resultant image

Posteroanterior Cephalogram

Image Field

It is used to survey the skull vault and primarily the facial bones for evidence of trauma, disease or developmental abnormality.

Fractures of the skull vault, investigation of frontal sinuses, conditions affecting the cranium (e.g. paget's disease, multiple myeloma, hyperparathyroidism), intracranial calcifications.

Position of Film

The cassette is placed perpendicular to the floor in a cassette holding device. The long-axis of the cassette is positioned vertically.

Position of Patients

The sagittal plane should be vertical and perpendicular to the film.

The head is tipped downward so that only the nose touches the film. The radiographic base line is at 10° with the film. The film is adjusted so that the lips are centered to the film.

Direction of Central Beam

It is directed at right angles to the film through the midsagittal plane, centered at the level of the bridge of the nose (Figs 2.52A to C).

Exposure parameter: kVp-84, mA-13, 1.5 seconds

Posteroanterior Skull

Image field

It is used to survey the skull vault and primarily the facial bones for evidence of trauma, disease or developmental abnormality.

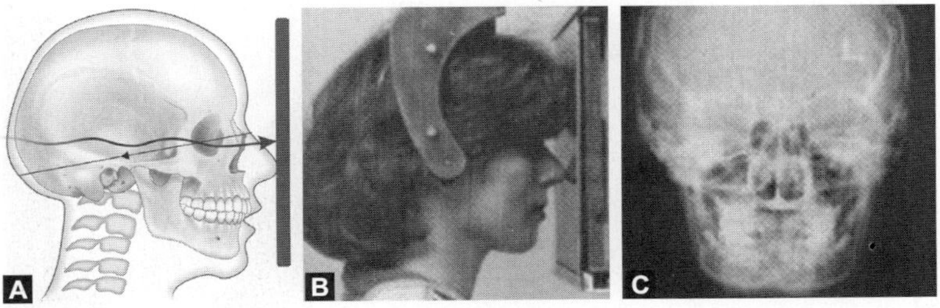

Figs 2.52A to C: PA cephalogram: Position of patients and cassette, direction of central beam and resultant image

Fractures of the skull vault, investigation of frontal sinuses, conditions affecting the cranium (e.g. paget's disease, multiple myeloma, hyperparathyroidism), intracranial calcifications.

Position of Film

The cassette is placed perpendicular to the floor in a cassette holding device. The long-axis of the cassette is positioned vertically.

Position of Patients

The sagittal plane should be vertical and perpendicular to the film. The head is tipped downward so that the forehead and nose touch the film. The radiographic base line is horizontal and perpendicular to the film.

The film is adjusted so that the lips are centered to the film.

Direction of Central Beam

It is directed at right angles to the film through the midsagittal plane through the occiput (Figs 2.53A and B).

Exposure parameter: kVp-65, mA-10, 2–3 seconds

Towne's Projection

Image Field

It is primarily used to observe the occipital area of the skull. The necks of the condyloid process can also be viewed.

Position of Film

The cassette is placed perpendicular to the floor in a cassette holding device. The long-axis of the cassette is positioned vertically.

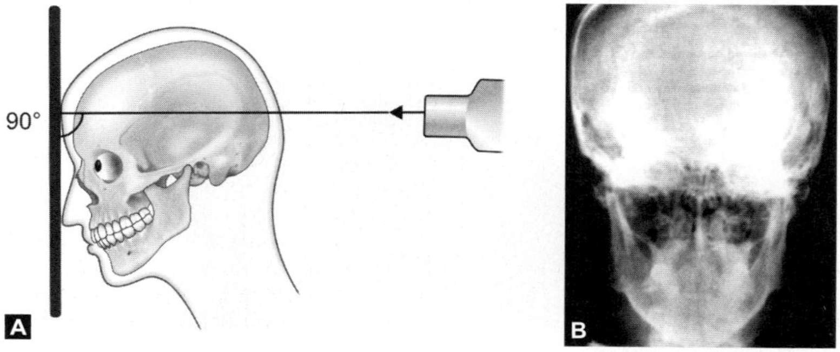

Figs 2.53A and B: PA skull projection: Position of patients and cassette, direction of central beam and resultant image

Position of Patients

This is an anteroposterior view, with the back of the patient's head touching the film. The canthomeatal line is perpendicular to the film.

Direction of Central Beam

It is directed at 30° to the canthomeatal line and passes through it at a point between the external auditory canals (Figs 2.54A and B).

Exposure parameter: kVp-65, mA-10, 2–3 seconds

Panoramic Imaging

Panoramic radiography also called pantomography or rotational radiography, is a radiographic technique for producing a single image of the facial structures that includes both maxillary and mandibular arches and their supporting structures.

The panoramic radiograph is often used as initial survey film that may provide the required insight or assist in determining the need for other projections.

Two basically different methods were initially proposed for panoramic radiography:

1. Use of intraoral source of radiation.
2. Use of an extra oralsource of radiation.

Intraoral Source of Radiation

Horst Beger of Dresden, Germany, invented the machine using intraoral source of radiation in 1943 during the World War II. This method employs an intraoral source of radiation.

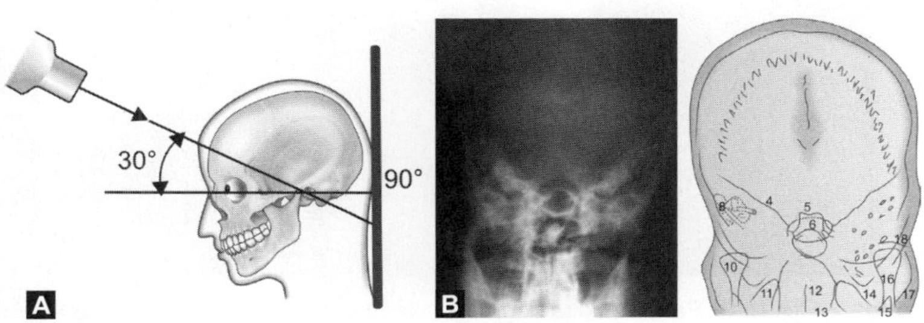

Figs 2.54A and B: Townes projection: Position of patients and cassette, direction of central beam and resultant image

The radiation is directed from inside the mouth through the jaws and exposes a film moulded to the outside of face of patient (Figs 2.55A to C) No screen or slow-speed films were used. The X-ray source, patient and film are stationary during the exposure.

Separate exposures were made for mandible and maxilla

- The machine required a very small focal spot(0.10–0.15 mm width), utilizing a tube current of 0.5–1.0 mA and a kilovoltage ranging from 40–80 kVp.
- Independently, Dr Walter Ott, a Swiss dentist, began developing an intraoral X-ray tube that could be inserted into patient's mouth. This method was later modified by Dr Sidney Blackman of England in 1960.

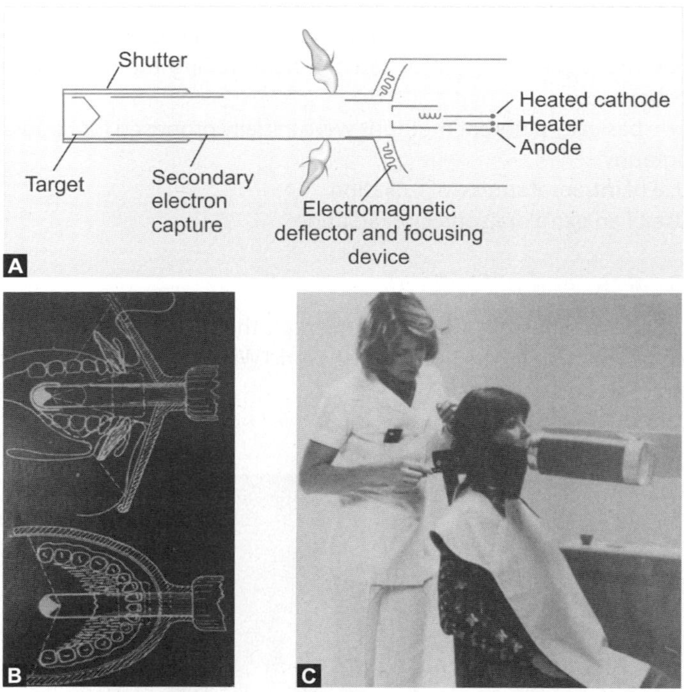

Figs 2.55A to C: Panoramic radiograph taken by using intraoral X-ray source

Extraoral Source of Radiation

Dr Numata H of Japan proposed and experimented this method of panoramic radiography for the first time in 1933. Twelve years later, Dr Paatero of Finland experimented and demonstrated the slit beam method of panoramic radiography in 1946. Both placed a curved film in mouth lingual to the teeth and used a slit or narrow X-ray beam (Fig. 2.56).

In Numata's model, X-ray beam rotated around the patient's jaws to expose the film.

While in Paatero's model, patient moved by means of a rotating chair and the X-ray source was stationary. This technique was called Parabolography.

In 1949, Paatero observed that panoramic radiographs could be taken with film placed extraorally. This technique was called Pantomography (Fig. 2.57).

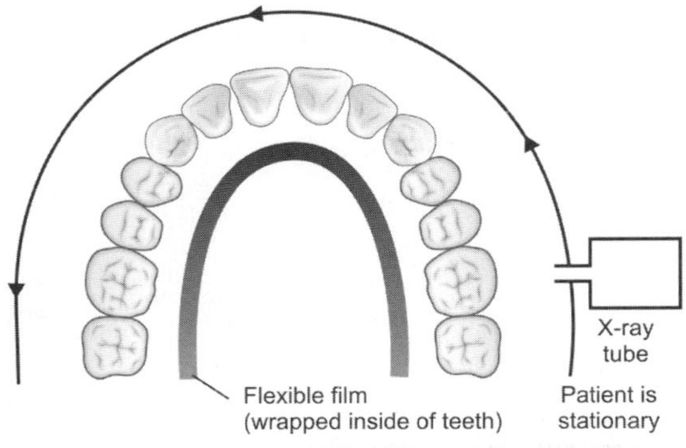

Fig. 2.56: Slit beam method of panoramic radiograph taken by placing the film lingual to teeth

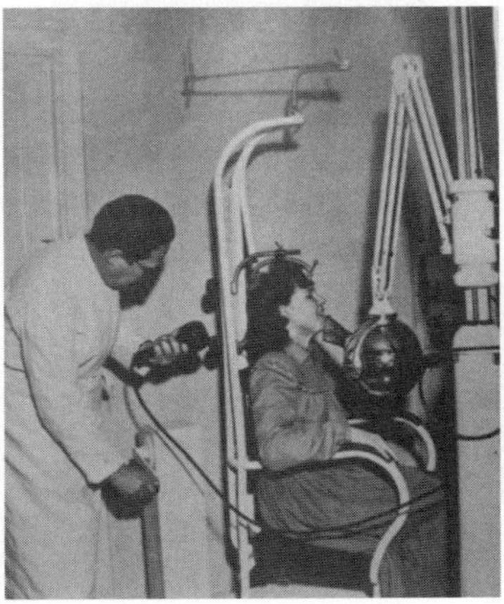

Fig. 2.57: Parabolography radiograph taken by placing the film extraorally

In early 1950, Dr Robert Nelson and John Kumpula, developed a technique called Panographic Radiography, in which a narrow beam of radiation was directed into a lead-backed curved film placed in mouth by means of a small film holder. Three radiographs were taken, one for each arch and a bite wing of crowns of both the arches (Figs 2.58A and B).

In 1950s, Panorex system developed in which the patient was kept stationary and the film and the tubehead were kept mobile. This method used two rotational axes.

In 1958, Paatero developed a new method called Orthoradial Jaw Pantomography, which used three axes of rotation. In this method, the patient remains stationary and the film rotating from the front of patient while the source rotating behind the neck of patient. Later on this name was changed to orthopantomography (Fig. 2.59).

In 1970s, Charles Morris and Don Hudson designed a unique panoramic unit called the Tomorex, which allowed the operator to take a panoramic radiograph of an injured or litter-borne patient (Fig. 2.60).

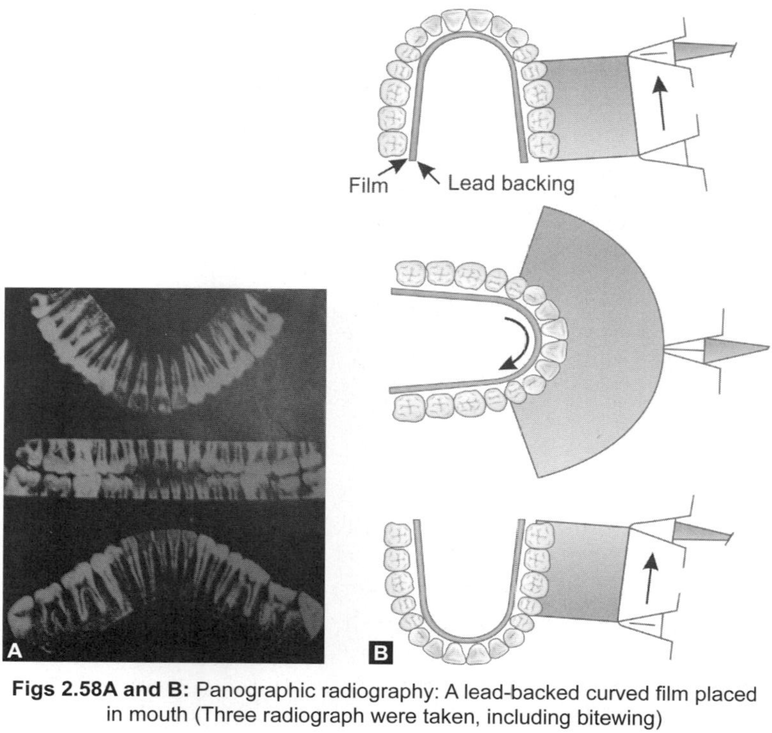

Figs 2.58A and B: Panographic radiography: A lead-backed curved film placed in mouth (Three radiograph were taken, including bitewing)

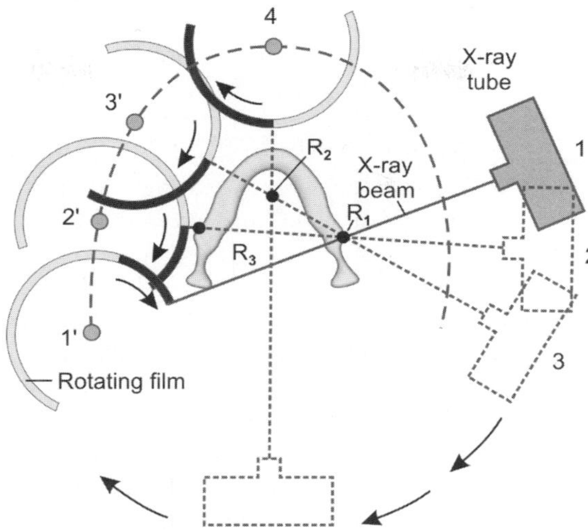

Fig. 2.59: Showing axis of rotation while taking orthopantomograph

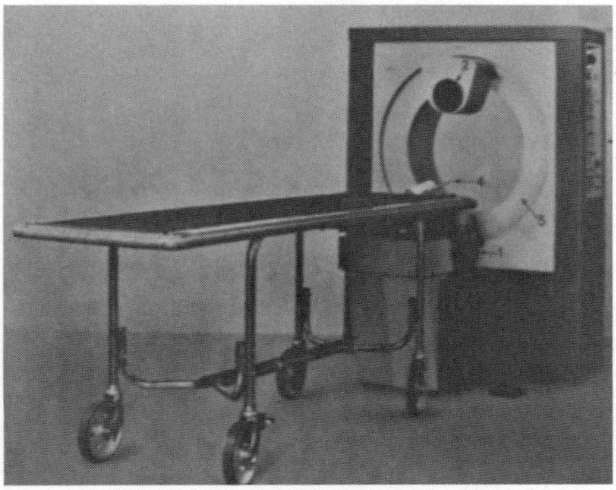

Fig. 2.60: Tomorex-Panoramic unit: Used for injured patients

Principles of Panoramic Image Formation

The principle of panoramic radiography was first described by Numata and independently by Paatero. The operation of panoramic machine can be understood by considering the following illustration:

- Two adjacent disks are rotating at the same speed in opposite directions as an X-ray beam passes through their center of rotation. Lead collimators in the shape of a slit are located at X-ray source and the film limit the central ray to a narrow vertical beam (Fig. 2.61).

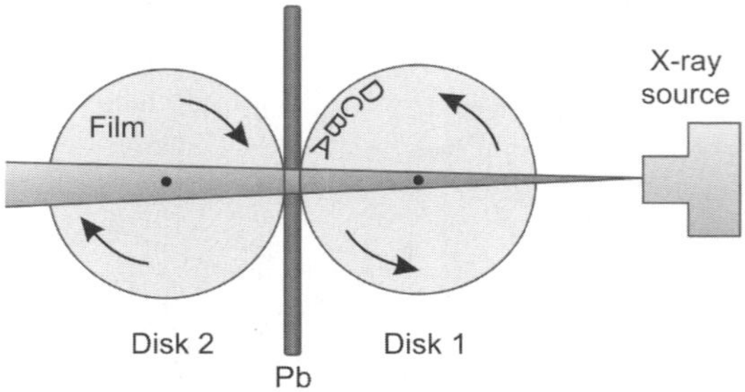

Fig. 2.61: Two disks moving with same speed and in opposite direction with X-ray beam passes through their center of rotation

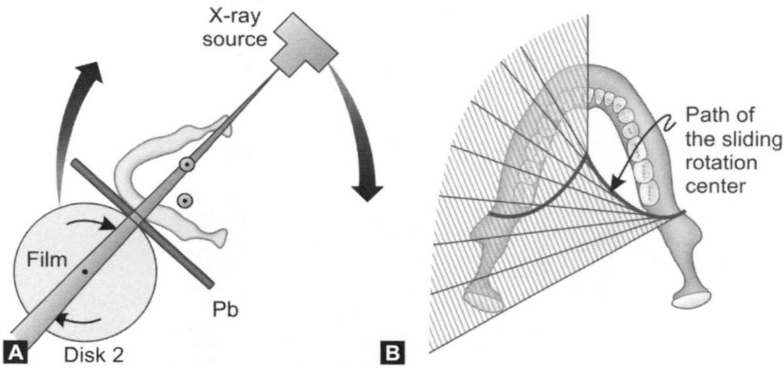

Figs 2.62A and B: Showing shifting of rotation center during movement of machine

- The objects are displayed sharply on the film because they are moving past the slit at the same rate as the film, which in effect causes their moving images to appear stationary in relation to the moving film.
- During the exposure cycle, the machine will automatically shift to other rotation centers. The movement of the film behind the slit is regulated to be the same as that of the central ray sweeping through the dental structures on the side of patient near the film (Figs 2.62A and B).

Focal Trough

Focal trough is a three-dimensional (3D) curved zone or image layer in which structures are reasonably well defined on panoramic radiograph (Fig. 2.63).

The width and the thickness is governed by factors which influence image definition:

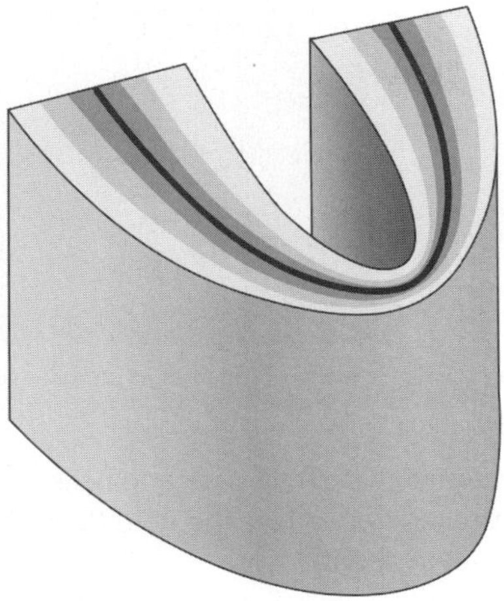

Fig. 2.63: Position of object in focal trough changes the size and shape of object

a. Arc path
b. Velocity of the film and X-ray tube head
c. Alignment of X-ray beam
d. Collimator width.

Shape of the focal trough varies with the brand of the equipment and extensive machine use can change the location of focal trough.

- As the position of the object is moved within the focal trough, the size and shape of the resultant image changes.

Patient Positioning and Head Alignment

- To obtain diagnostically useful panoramic radiographs, it is necessary to properly position patient's head in focal trough
- Dental appliances, earrings, necklaces, hairpins and any other metallic objects in head and neck region should be removed
- Patients should be instructed not to move during the procedure
- The maxilla and mandible can be placed in position by using bite block
- Midsagittal plane must be centered in focal trough
- The occlusal plane is aligned at the angle 20°–30° below the horizontal
- The chin is positioned so that the line from tragus of ear to outer canthus of eye is parallel with the floor.

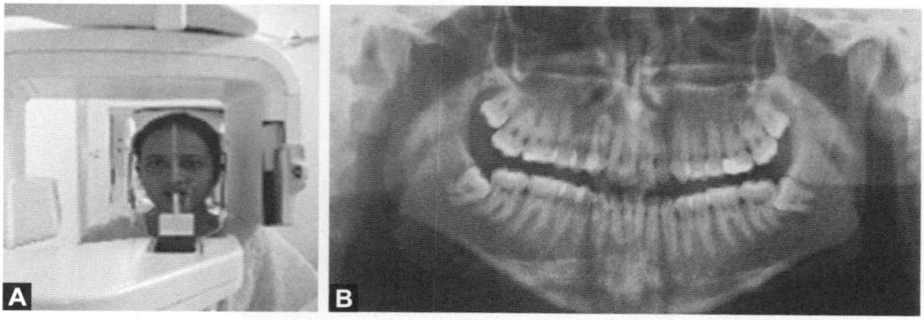

Figs 2.64A and B: Position of patients in panoramic machine

- Patients are positioned with their back and neck extended
- Patients are instructed to swallow and hold the tongue on the roof of the mouth (Figs 2.64A and B).

Indications

As a substitute for full mouth intraoral periapical radiographs

- Evaluation of mixed dentition in children
- To assist and assess the patient for and during orthodontic treatment
- To establish the site and size of the lesion like cysts, tumors and developing anomaly in the body or rami of mandible and maxilla
- As a guiding tool before surgical procedures such as extraction of impacted tooth, enucleation of cyst, etc.
- Detection of fractures of mandible and mid facial regions after trauma.
- For follow up of treatment, progress of a pathology or tracing healing of bone
- Investigation of temporomandibular joint
- Study of antrum, esp. floor, posterior and anterior wall of antrum
- As an overall view of the alveolar bone levels in periodontal disease
- Assessment of underlying bone before constructing complete or partial dentures
- Evaluating the height of bone before insertion of implants.

Advantages

- Simple procedure requiring very little patient compliance
- Convenient for the patients
- Useful in patients with trismus and gagging problems
- Time required is minimum as compared to full mouth intraoral radiographs

- Patient's dose is relatively low
- Act as valuable visual aid in patient education
- Maximum areas of maxilla and mandible and midfacial region are visible on a single radiograph
- It allows for assessment of the presence and position of unerupted teeth in orthodontic treatment
- All parameters are standardized and repetitive images can be taken, on recall visits for comparative and research purposes
- Useful for mass screening
- Helps in localization of objects or pathology in conjunction with a topographic occlusal view or an intraoral periapical view.

Disadvantages

- Areas of diagnostic interest outside the focal trough may be poorly visualized
- Comparatively panoramic radiograph is of a poor diagnostic quality, in terms of magnification, poor definition and loss of details
- There is overlapping of teeth in the bicuspid area of maxilla and mandible
- The density of spine, especially in short necked people can cause lack of clarity in the central portion of the film
- Number of radiopaque and radiolucent areas may be present because of the superimposition of real/double or ghost images and due to soft tissue shadows and air spaces
- Due to prescribed rotation, patients with facial asymmetry cannot be X-rayed with satisfaction
- Artifacts are easily misinterpreted and are more commonly seen
- OPG shows an oblique, rather than true lateral view of the condylar heads and hence, the joint space cannot be accurately assessed
- The cost of the machine is very high.

Darkroom Techniques

- Reduction in darkroom lighting is required as exposed panoramic films are more sensitive to light
- The filter (ML-2) which is used while processing intraoral films transmits the light of such wavelength that can fog panoramic films. Hence, a Kodak GBX-2 filter can be installed with a 15 watt bulb at least 4 feet from working area

- Panoramic films should be developed either manually or in automatic processor using manufacturer's recommendations

Dose Reduction

- There is low dose exposure to patient with panoramic radiographs due to use of intensifying screens
- The dose of patient through one panoramic radiograph is equivalent to 4 bite wing radiographs
- As the kVp cannot be reduced below 65, to reduce patient's dose, filters can be used, e.g. Lanex screen.

3 Tomography

Radiology began as a medical subspecialty in first decade of the 1900s after the discovery of X-ray by Professor Roentgen. The development of radiology grew at a good pace until World War II. Extensive use of X-ray imaging during the second World War, and the advent of the digital computer and new imaging modalities like tomography, computed tomography (CT), nuclear medicine imaging, ultrasound, magnetic resonance imaging (MRI) have combined to create an explosion of diagnostic imaging technique. The growing interest in digital imaging has resulted for number of reasons. These include elimination of the dark room; elimination of hard copy, thereby decreasing storage needs up to 90% when compared with film. In addition, the value of the digital image can be extended through the use of software algorithms. The digital process quantizes the image into discrete two-dimensional (2D) areas (pixels) or three-dimensional (3D) volumes (voxels).The pixels and voxels can be described by a dimension (height and width for pixel; height, width, and thickness for a voxel) location, and a value (gray scale or color).

In most types of digital radiography, electromagnetic energy (X-radiation) is converted to an electrical charge by an X-ray sensor. The X-ray sensor includes charge-coupled devices (CCDs), charged phosphor, amorphous silicon, and amorphous selenium. CCDs are small sensors like those found in video cameras. To determine the suitability of digital imaging as an alternative to conventional imaging methods, the most important criteria that must be considered are its spatial resolution and gray-scale resolving power. Although gray-scale resolution is determined by the number of bits/pixels (number of gray levels). Although spatial resolution depends on the relative difference between the number of pixels available in the image-capturing device and the size of the object being imaged. Finally, digital imaging offers additional advantages since the imaging data can be enhanced by being processed through desired algorithm to achieve specific imaging objectives. All these advance imaging techniques are has been successfully used for maxillofacial region evaluation, as per the requirements.

TOMOGRAPHY

In plain film studies, there is superimposition of different structures; to avoid this several radiographic techniques have been developed with the purpose of demonstrating individual body areas distinct from the surrounding anatomic structures.

Tomographic methods used commonly in dentistry can be divided into conventional tomography and computed tomography. Conventional tomographic techniques consist of common components like X-ray tube, X-ray film, and a ridge-connecting bar, which rotates around a fixed fulcrum. The type of tube motion influences whether a technique is termed linear tomography or pluridirectional tomography (Figs 3.1A and B).

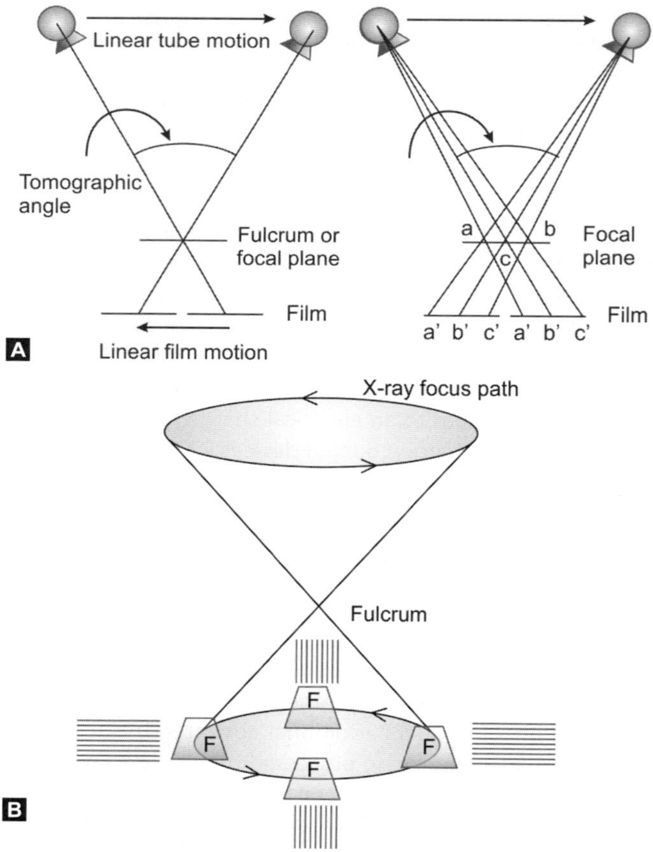

Figs 3.1A and B: (A) Linear tomographic motion showing tube and film movement; (B) Plane of interest at the level of fulcrum

During linear tomography the radiographic tube moves in one direction, the film moves in the opposite direction, and the system remains stationary. The level of fulcrum is represented in the patient as the layer of interest where the anatomic structures are in sharp focus. All the point above and below this plane are blurred. The thickness of this layer of interest is determined by the degrees in the tomographic angle.

The section thickness or cut is inversely proportional to the tomographic angle. Thus, the larger the tomographic angle, the thinner the section. The more complex tube movement like circular, elliptical, figure-eight, hypocycloidal, and trispiral have been designed to provide a more uniform blurring of the objects with a more consistent cut or section thickness. The resulting imaging may be easier to interprete because there are no streaks and the overall image contrast is improved (Fig. 3.2).

One of the primary applications for conventional tomography in dentistry is the diagnostic imaging of the temporomandibular joint (TMJ) complex. Tomographic studies in the lateral and coronal planes demonstrate osseous components of the joint, whereas arthrotomographic examinations provide information about the status of the soft tissue like intra-articular disk (Figs 3.3 and 3.4).

Most conventional tomographic studies of the TMJ include lateral projection in close and open positions exposed at an angle that corrects for the angle of condyle relative to the horizontal axis, so that the TMJ is perpendicular to the film during a lateral tomographic cut and parallel to it's for a frontal or coronal tomogram. Corrected coronal tomographic images

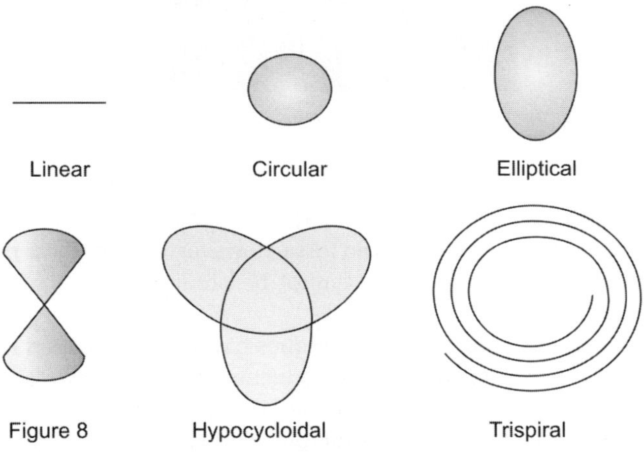

Fig. 3.2: Type of movement for pluridirectional tomography

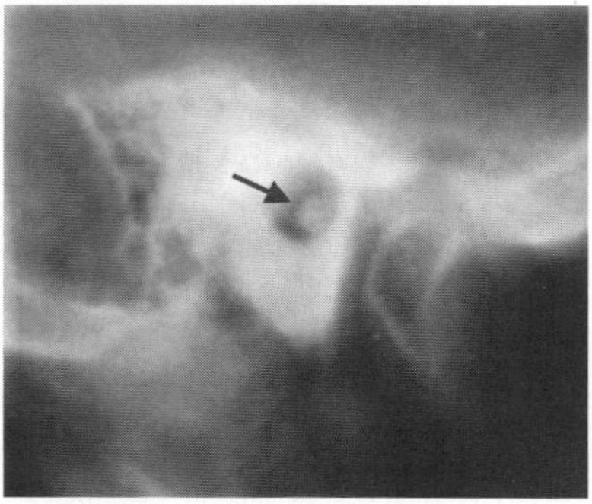

Fig. 3.3: Linear tomographic image: Corrected lateral view of TMJ complex

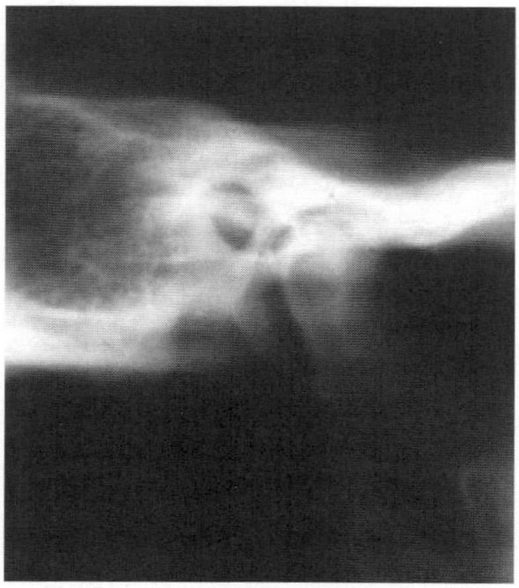

Fig. 3.4: Pluridirectional tomography image with octospiral motion

provide additional information about the condylar head and glenoid fossa. Because corrected lateral tomograms demonstrate the location of the condyle relative to the glenoid fossa, however, that condylar position is so variable that disk position cannot be predicted reliably from the tomographic images.

A number of arthrographic techniques have been described that use tomography before and after the introduction of contrast media into the joint spaces. Scout tomograms may be taken prior to the arthrographic procedure to visualize osseous structures and condylar position, and to select the image layer for the arthrotomogram.

Another important dental application for conventional tomography is the presurgical radiographic examination of proposed implant site. Tomographic images demonstrate individual implant site characteristics such as proximity to the surrounding anatomic structures, the available vertical length and horizontal width to appropriate implant, characteristic of the alveolar crest.

A linear tomographic technique can be used to determine the buccolingual relationship of impacted mandibular third molar to the inferior alveolar canal prior to extraction, and also can be used prior to endodontic surgery to demonstrate the proximity of mandibular molar root apices to the inferior alveolar canal.

4 Computed Tomography

Computed tomography (CT) is a radiographic technique that blends the concepts of thin-layer radiography (tomography) with computer synthesis of the image (computed). X-ray beam attenuation measurements are made in a 360° circle around the part of the patients' body being scanned (Fig. 4.1). These measurements are then fed into a computer, which construct an image from them. The image then can be displayed on a video monitor, reformatted into other planes in two- or three-dimensions, adjusted for optimum viewing of bone or soft tissue, stored on magnetic tape or optical disk. Once the initial CT scan is performed, all of the subsequent image manipulation can be performed on a computer after the patient has left. But before reviewing the uses of CT in dentistry, clinicians need to understand the basic principles of CT image formation, including the terminology used to various aspects of the image.

The equipment needed to produce a CT scan consist of a donut-shaped scanning gantry, which contains the X-ray source, detectors and electronic measuring devices, a motorized table used to position the patient within the gantry, X-ray power supplies and controls a computer and viewing devices such as video monitors. Image can be filmed from the monitor by special slave imager cameras. Image data can be stored on magnetic tapes or disks (Fig. 4.2).

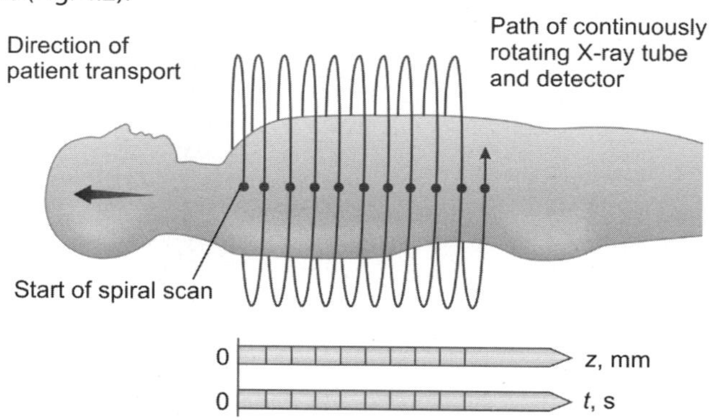

Fig. 4.1: Direction of patient moving and path of rotation of X-ray tube

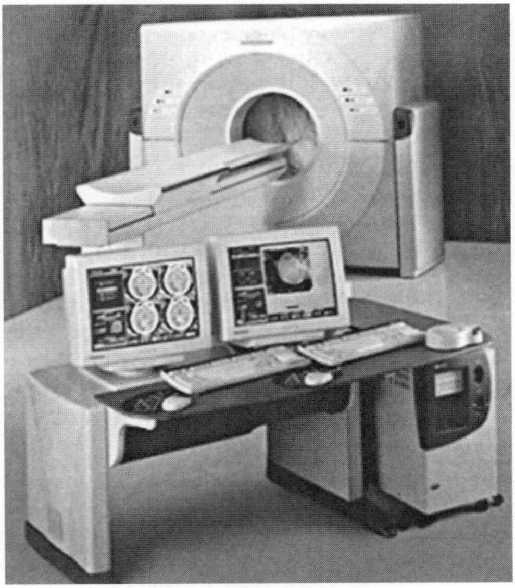

Fig. 4.2: Advance CT scanner

In the early days of CT scanning, the X-ray beam and detector moved linearly on either side of the patient's head, collecting the attenuation data that would eventually form the image. At the end of each linear scan, the gantry would rotate 1degree and the scan would be repeated, over and over again until 180° of rotation had occurred (Fig. 4.3).

Equipment improvements over the years include the use of multiple detectors and elimination of the translate phase of X-ray beam movement by using a fan-shaped beam to cover a larger area. In many modern machines today the detectors, either scintillation crystals or xenon gas, are arranged in either a rotating arc opposite the X-ray generator or a 360° array around the patient's body. During a scan, the X-ray tube rotates around the patient once for each slice, thus reducing the time of the entire scan from the original 30 minites or so to 2 second per slice (Fig. 4.4).

The X-ray beam attenuation data are collected in a grid pattern called a matrix. Each square in the matrix is made up a pixel, which represents the X-ray attenuation of a small finite volume of tissue. The area of tissue scanned and the size of the matrix determine the size of the pixel. Typical matrix sizes in CT are 256x256 or 512x512 pixels. The smaller the size of each individual pixel, the finer will be the overall image resolution (Fig. 4.5).

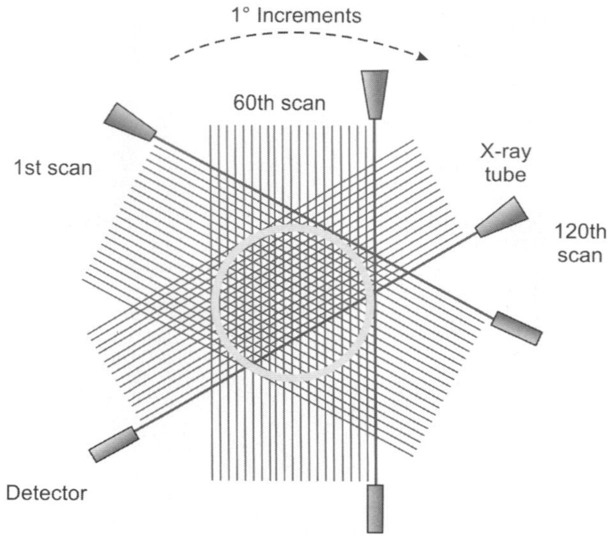

Fig. 4.3: First generation CT scanner. Beam translate through patient then rotate 1 degree for next scan

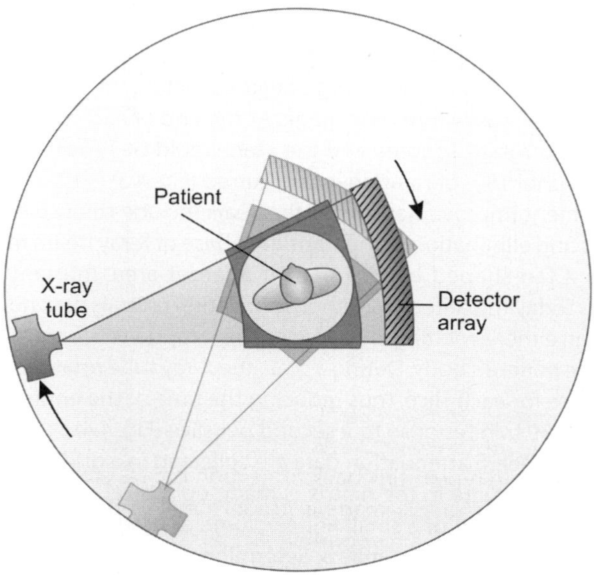

Fig. 4.4: Fan beam scanner. X-ray tube and detector array rotated around the patient ones for each scan slice

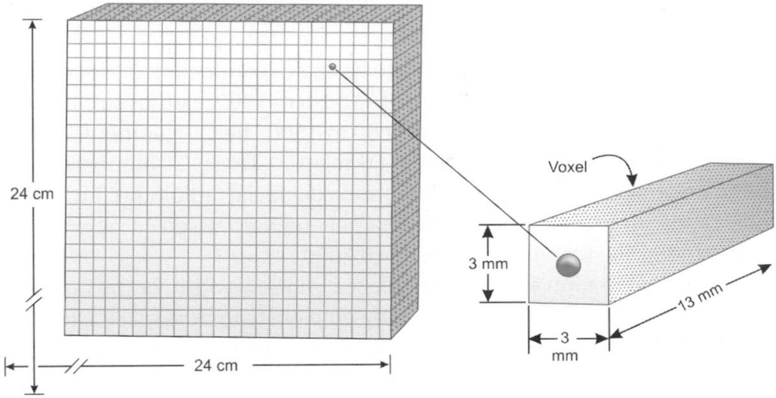

Fig. 4.5: Computer matrix, pixel and voxel

The CT image is made up a series of slice, each of which represents the anatomy of layer of soft tissue. The slice thickness is chosen by the operator. The finer detail can be obtained with thinner slice. In clinical practice, abdominal and other body CT imaging is performed at 10 mm thick slice; whereas head CT scans are usually made with 3 mm slice. Three-dimensional (3D) reformatting generally requires slice thickness of 1–1.5 mm. Thinner the slice, the more slice are needed to cover the tissue and the higher the radiation dose to the patient.

The data that are collected by the detectors are based on the attenuation of the X-ray beam by all the tissues in the path of the beam. If the intensity of the X-ray beam when it enters the patient is of a certain magnitude, say 10 unit, and the intensity when it hits the detector is only 4 units, then the tissue has absorbed 6 unit of X-ray. To produce an image from these data we need to know, how the attenuation was distributed throughout the tissue.

The attenuation measurement is apportioned equally among all the voxels in path of the X-ray beam. As data from 360° around the patient are available, one can repeat this back projection process for each detector. Each pixel in the resultant image is proportional to the sum of the rays projected through its corresponding voxels. To minimize artifacts, the computer dose some modification or filtering of the data to produce an image that is a close approximation of the attenuation characteristics of the object.

Once all the calculations are performed, the results are in the form of a pixel map of attenuation number, each of which has a physical meaning. For example, water is set by convention to have a CT number of -0 (Hounsfield Unit) whereas fat has a CT number of –100; air –1000; various soft tissues, from about 12 to 80; and bone, from 80 to 1500.The CT Number for most biologic tissues are in the range of –50 to +100. These CT numbers must be transformed into an image. In dentomaxillofacial radiology CT number may range up to 3000 or more for enamel and hard tissue CT number for dense metal like titanium may be up to 7000 HU.

At the video monitor, one can select a window width, or the range of CT numbers that will be represented by pure white to pure black. One also can select a window level, or the CT number, that will correspond to the middle of the continuum from white to black. This is similar to adjusting the contrast and brightness controls on a television. To produce image variation, one simply alters window width and level on the monitor.

ADVANTAGES OF COMPUTED TOMOGRAPHY

Superimposition of Structures

When a conventional radiograph is made, all structures in the path of the X-ray beam will show up on the radiograph. This is not the problem for image of the axial skeleton, such as arms and legs, because the bone are thin and limb can be moved away from the rest of body, thus allowing the beam to be directed from multiple angles if needed. The head, however, has much more complicated anatomy, especially in the maxillofacial region and cranial base.

CT solves this problem of superimposition by allowing the clinician to view a series of thin sections, 1.5–10 mm thick depending on anatomic region, completely through the area of interest. Each layer can be visualized unobstructed by other anatomic features typically, all the layers are viewed sequentially so the clinician can determine the full extent of the pathology.

Image Acquisition in Cross-sectional or Other Planes

In conventional plain or tomographic radiography, the view desired to demonstrate the pathology, places the film behind the body part, and directs the beam through the structure of interest. Standard frontal and lateral images are not too difficult to obtain in most area of the body. Cross-sectional image, however, cannot be made many body regions because it is not possible to place the film and beam in the correct position. With CT, however axial or cross-sectional image are made routinely because of the arrangement of the detectors around the patient's body and the computer processing of the detector signals. Once the data are collected and processed, an operator sitting at a console can reformat the images into desired planes.

Soft Tissue Imaging

Plain radiographs demonstrate calcified structures very well but provide little information regarding soft tissues because of the screen systems to record X-ray attenuation differences of less than 2%.

CT imaging, however, is much more effective at separating subtle tissues contrast differences (as low as 0.5%) and thus can be used to differentiate not only soft tissue from bone, but also various types of soft tissue from each other.

When even more information is required concerning the soft tissues, an intravenous contrast agent can be used, which will accentuated the differences in tissue because the agent is concentrated in tissue with high vascularity.

Adjustment of Radiographic Contrast

Once a plain radiograph is made, there is little that can be done without a computer to alter the contrast or otherwise enhance the image. With CT, however, the operator at the console can adjust the contrast and brightness, similarly to adjusting the controls on a television set. In addition operator can emphasize the contrasts in bone (make a so-called "bone window") or in soft tissue (soft tissue window) depending on the nature of the pathology being evaluated.

Early Diagnosis

Disease processes may be detected at an earlier stage than is possible with other techniques and lesions may be detected in areas, which are difficult to assess with conventional imaging.

DISADVANTAGES OF CT SCAN

Most of the survey indicated that there is fairly wide ranges of radiation doses used in performing a CT scan of the head, with the majority of machines producing a mid-skull dose of between 34 mGy and 55 mGy (3.4–5.5 rad). This can be compared to a mean entrance exposure of 5.3 mGy (530 mrad) for posteroanterior or townes view skull radiograph.

Although CT is effective in disease detection and localization, the characterization of lesions is more difficult, since many have similar attenuation characteristics. For example, it may not be possible to distinguish fibrotic masses from benign or malignant neoplasm on the basis of their CT appearance alone.

The other main disadvantages of CT are the capital cost of the equipment and the fact that it employs ionizing radiation. CT is used with care around radiosensitive structures such as the eye, or in children and young people, and only for over-riding indications in pregnant women.

Therapeutic Uses

A wide range of percutaneous therapeutic procedures are performed under CT control. The most common technique is CT guided biopsy; aspiration for diagnostic cytology or cutting needle biopsy for histological diagnosis can be undertaken in virtually any area of the body. CT-guided drainage can also be used in the treatment of most deep seated abscesses and other pathological fluid collection. Guided neurolysis, tumor lysis by alcohol injection, and laser therapy can also be under CT control.

Uses of Computed Tomography in Dentistry

A very important use of CT in dentistry is the evaluation of the presence and extent of clinically suspected pathology in the head and neck, including tumors, cysts and infections. When the lesion extended into the neck or the maxillary sinus or anywhere in soft tissues in the head, however, CT imaging is useful in determining the extent of the pathology. This type of information is invaluable for treatment planning.

Another major use of CT in dentistry is the determination of the location and displacement of facial fractures in maxillofacial region.

If the CT scan is performed with thin (1.5 mm) continuous slices, the data can be reformatted into a 3D image that can be rotated on the video screen to demonstrate the anatomy and pathology from all angles, which help in the reconstruction of jaws or joints. With some 3D software algorithms, individual bones and tumors can be disarticulated from the rest of the anatomy to increase visualization of specified structures.

CT is the best technique for imaging the TMJ. CT is also useful for evaluation of bony changes in patients with implants in the TMJ. There have been reports of foreign body granulomas associated with these implant causing perforation through the glenoid fossa into the middle cranial fossa.

CT is the best technique for determine the presence of such a perforation. Another use for CT scanning in dentistry is for the evaluation of the jaws of patient for dental implants. After thin section axial CT scans are made through the mandible or maxilla, dedicated software programs are used to reformat the data into a panoramic type image as well as cross-sectional images perpendicular to a curved plane through the arch. In this way, buccal-lingual width of the jaw as well as the location of anatomical features such as the mandibular canal or maxillary sinus can be determined.

CT Guided Biopsy Techniques

Guided biopsy is used widely in many areas of the body, primarily as a method of obtaining material for histological or microbiological examination that would otherwise only be available by open operation. It is also used increasingly in situations where simple percutaneous fine-needle biopsy is possible, but cannot be relied upon to sample and the area of biopsy is not confirmed. Examples would include small or impalpable lesions, patchy involvement by a diffuse process, or circumstances where a complicated angulation of the biopsy device is required to reach the target lesion. The particular method used to perform such biopsy is dependent not only upon the clinical circumstances, but upon the preferences of the radiologist.

CT guided techniques enable a two-dimensional (2D) image with skin markers to be produced, from which the entry point, angulations, and depth of insertion of the biopsy device may be electronically planned. The main disadvantage is that, as the biopsy device is advanced toward the lesion, the procedure must be interrupted, and repeat scanning performed, at intervals which depend upon the anatomic complexity. Sophisticated software programmers are available to plan a 3D approach to lesions where direct access is hindered by bony or important structures.

Contraindications

1. Patients with allergy to dye or shellfish.
2. Patients those are pregnant.
3. Patients with unstable vital signs.
4. Patients that are very obese (over 300 lbs).
5. Patients with metal implants or pacemakers.
6. Since the Barium interferes the image, patients that have recently had imaging techniques that use barium.

Cone-beam Computed Tomography

Role of cone-beam computed tomography (CBCT), for dental and maxillofacial diagnostic osseous tasks has been rapidly developed as an alternative to conventional CT for assessment of the maxillofacial pathology specially TMJ. CBCT results in images of CT-like quality, yet is made with less expensive equipment and components, shorter patient examination time, and much lower radiation dose than required for conventional CT.

CBCT provides images that can be reconstructed in planes parallel or perpendicular to the long axis of the condyle instead of the true anatomic coronal and sagittal planes. This results in high quality images of the bony components in all planes. Because the patients are positioned in a relatively natural head position, the TMJ positional relationships can be more accurately evaluated than in a CT examination, where the patient is supine position (Figs 4.6 and 4.7).

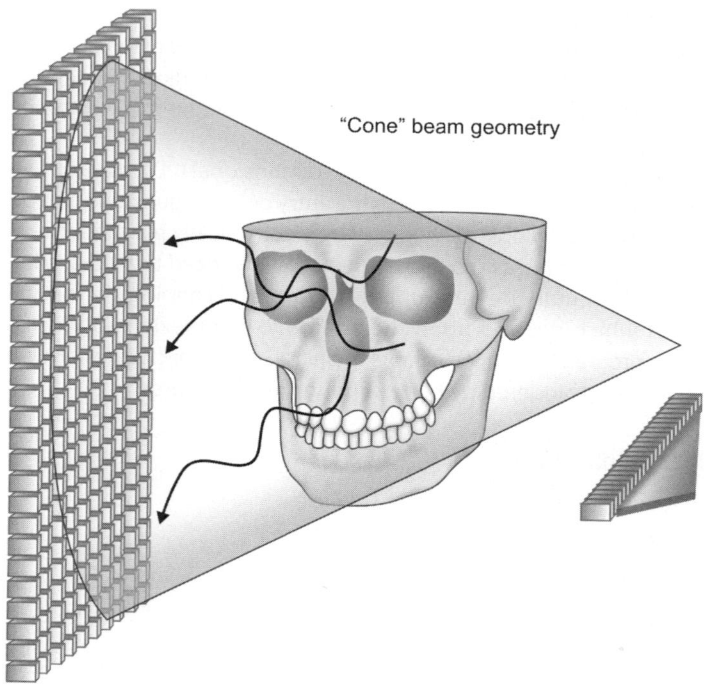

Fig. 4.6: Geometry of cone beam

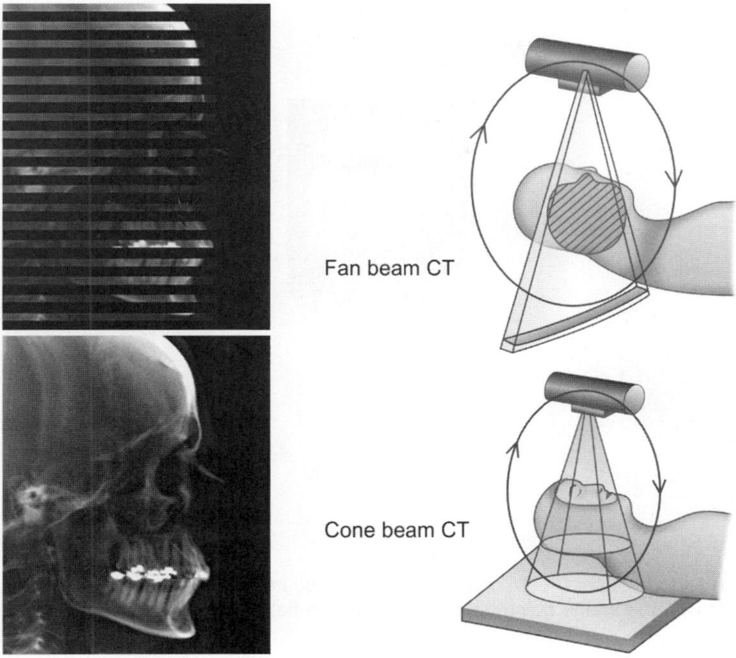

Fig. 4.7: Position of patients for fan beam CT and cone beam CT

CBCT Image Production

There are four components to CBCT image acquisition: (1) X-ray generation, (2) Image detection, (3) Image reconstruction, and (4) Image display. Cone-beam scanners are based on a cone-shaped beam of X-rays rotating around the object of interest giving a volume of data, using a 2D extended digital array as an area detector (Fig. 4.8).

The technique involves a single 360° scan in which the X-ray source and reciprocating area detector synchronously move around the patient's head, which is stabilized with a head holder. At certain degree intervals, single projection images, known as 'basis' images, are acquired. These are similar to lateral cephalometric radiographic images, each slightly offset from one another. This series of basis projection images is referred to as the projection data. Software programmes incorporating sophisticated algorithms, including back-filtered projection, are applied to these image data to generate a 3D volumetric dataset, and can be used to provide primary reconstruction images in three orthogonal planes (axial, sagittal and coronal), as well as three-dimensionally.

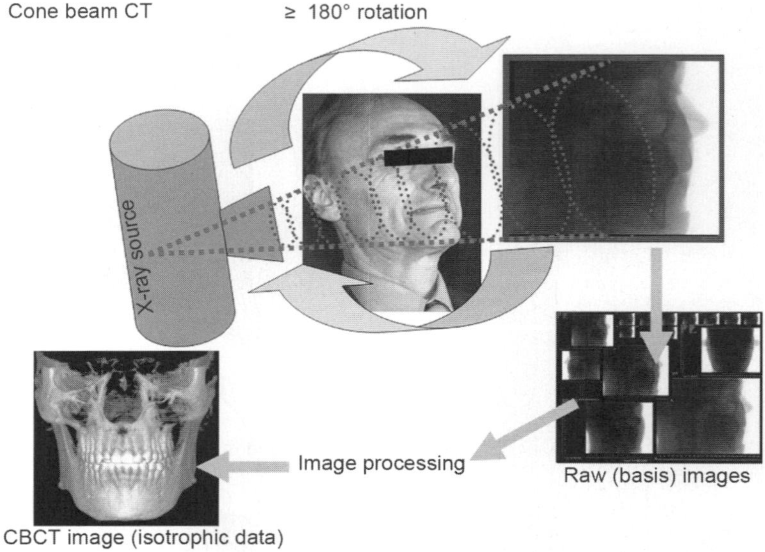

Fig. 4.8: Cone-beam CT – a cone-shaped X-ray beam rotates around a stationary patient with the image being detected by either a flat panel detector or an image intensifier

Clinical Applications of Cone-beam Imaging

Cone-beam CT is an exciting new addition to the imaging armamentarium which can be utilized to investigate the head and neck. It has the potential to transform practically all aspects of dental imaging. It offers an alternative to the need for complicated interpretative reasoning currently used, e.g. in parallax techniques for location of unerupted teeth. For ectopic, palatally placed maxillary canines parallax techniques have been shown to have a sensitivity of 69%, using a vertical technique, and 88% for horizontal parallax, but for buccally displaced canines these sensitivity figures both drop to 63%. In view of these figures and with the advent of cone-beam imaging, which gives so much more detail, perhaps the dose/benefit ratio needs to be reappraised. The 3D nature of the data obtained allows easy visualization of structures in the complex maxillofacial environment. The potential scope of clinical applications for cone-beam imaging is vast and currently has been shown to be particularly useful in the following dental and maxillofacial areas (Figs 4.9 and 4.10).

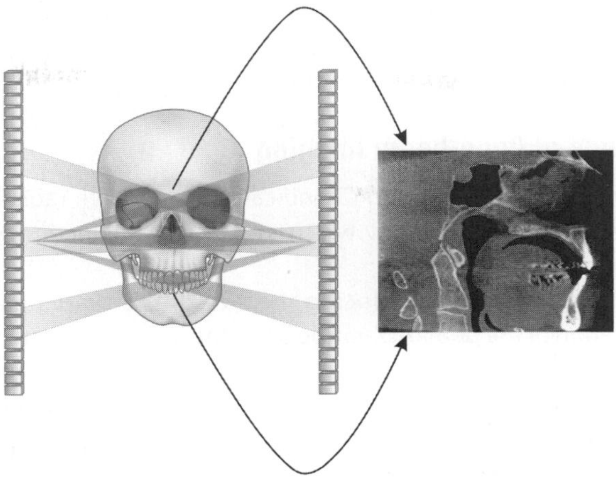

Fig. 4.9: Cone-beam application for dental and maxillofacial areas

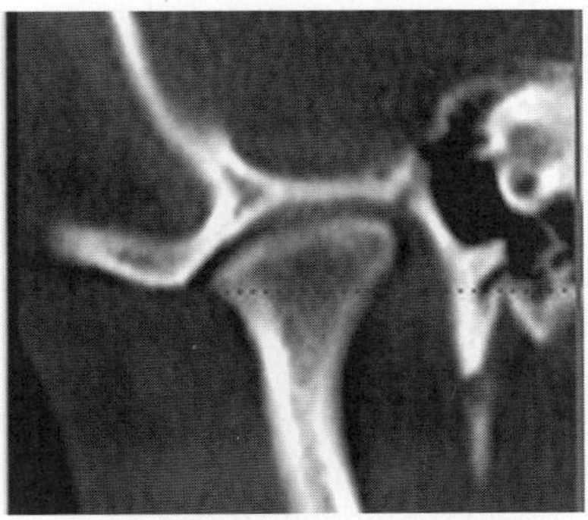

Fig. 4.10: CBCT image of temporomandibular joint

- Investigation of various jaw pathology includes cysts, tumors and fibro-osseous lesions
- Investigation of the paranasal sinuses diseases
- Investigation of the bony components of the TMJ
- Pre- and post-implant assessment
- Orthodontic assessment, both dental development and skeletal base relationship
- Assessment of wisdom teeth, in particular their relationship to the inferior dental canal
- Evaluation of facial trauma.

In addition, it provides the capability to visualize anything three-dimensionally; from anatomical tooth anomalies as, e.g. in endodontic cases, to the composition of periodontal defects.

Advantages of Cone-beam Imaging

- *Dose reduction*: Cone-beam CT indicates an effective radiation dose between 0.035 and 0.10 mSv, which is up to a 98% reduction compared to conventional CT.
- *X-ray beam limitation*: Reducing the size of the irradiated area by collimation of the primary X-ray beam to the area of interest minimizes the radiation dose.
- *Rapid scan times*: All the basis images are acquired in a single rotation; scan time is quick, varying between 10 and 40 seconds. Fast scan times also result in fewer artifacts.
- *Image accuracy*: The volumetric dataset comprises a 3-D block of smaller cuboid units, known as voxels, each representing a specific degree of X-ray absorption. The size of these voxels determines the resolution of the image ranging from 0.4 mm to as low as 0.125 mm.

Disadvantages of CBCT

- CBCT technology has limitations related to the "cone beam" projection geometry, detector sensitivity and contrast resolution
- These parameters create an inherent image "noise" that reduces image clarity
- Unable to record soft tissue contrast at the relatively low dosages applied for maxillofacial imaging
- Image degradation due to motion artifact
- Cone-beam technology based on an image intensifier may allow the periphery of the image to be distorted
- Radiological interpretation can be difficult when using a smaller field of view.

5 Sialography

The diagnostic imaging of salivary gland disease may be undertaken to differentiate inflammatory processes from neoplastic disease, distinguish diffuse disease from focal suppurative disease, identify and localize sialoliths, and demonstrate ductal morphology. In addition, diagnostic imaging attempts to determine the anatomic location of a tumor, differentiate benign from malignant disease, and demonstrate the relationship between a mass and adjacent anatomic structure and aid in the selection of biopsy sites.

Sialography is a radiographic technique in which a radiopaque contrast agent is infused into the ductal system of a salivary gland prior to imaging with plain films, fluoroscopy, panoramic radiography, tomography, or computed tomography (CT). Sialography provides a straightforward demonstration of the ductal system.

It is useful diagnostic adjunct to reveal location and integrity of salivary glands, thus indicating the presence of diseases that changes internal architecture.

Indications for Sialography

1. Evaluation of chronic inflammatory diseases and ductal pathosis.
2. Detection of calculus or calculi or foreign bodies.
3. To find out the destruction of gland secondary to obstructing calculi or foreign bodies.
4. Diagnosis of recurrent swellings and inflammatory processes.
5. Demonstration of a tumor and the determination of its location, size and origin and whether the radiographs suggest a benign or malignant-lesion.
6. Detection and portrayal of fistulae, diverticula's or strictures.
7. Selection of site for biopsy.
8. Outline of the plane of facial nerve as a guide in planning a biopsy or dissection.
9. Detection of residual stone or stones, residual tumor, fistula or stenoses or retention cysts following prior simple lithotomy or other surgical procedures.

Contraindications for Sialography

1. Patients with known sensitivity to iodine compounds and patients who have experienced severe asthmatic attacks or anaphylaxis following use of iodine compounds in a prior radiographic examination should not be considered subjects for this technique.
2. In case of acute inflammation of the salivary gland system sialography is contraindicated.
3. The administration and retention of iodinated contrast material may interfere with subsequent thyroid function tests, such function studies, if required, should be performed prior to the use of sialography.

CONTRAST MEDIA

The salivary glands being soft-tissue structures are not visible radiographically. They are made visible by the technique of sialography which involves the use of retrograde filling of the luminal system with radiopaque contrast media. Rankow RM and Polayes IM (1976) described two types of contrast media for studies on salivary ductal system.

I. Lipid or fat soluble contrast media which are again classified as:

1. Iodized Oils

   For example: ethiodal, lipiodal, lipiodal ultra-fluid (UF), T-odochloral.

   Properties:

   a. They have an iodine content ranging from 37–41% w/w.
   b. They have a specific gravity ranging from 1.28–1.36 at 150 c.
   c. They are highly viscous, with their viscosity ranging from 80-100 centipose.

   Advantages:

   a. They produce a satisfactory degree of radiographic opacifications with sustained opacity making possible to study the post evacuation phase.
   b. It produces sharper visualization with good resolution of the most peripheral ducts.

   Disadvantages:

   a. It produces greater degree of discomfort to the patient.
   b. They tend to retain within the glands when overfilled and cause an inflammatory reaction together with granuloma formation and subsequent fibrosis.

c. It causes clouding of the gland due to greater amounts of contrast medium within the lining of fine ducts and capillaries. Verhoeven JW and Utrechi (1984) in study of contrast agents recommended Lipoidal UF as the best among oily contrast media available.

2. Water—insoluble organic iodine compounds
For example, pentopaque, myodil

II. Water soluble contrast media (Sinographin)
for example: Hypaque 50, Urograffin, Hypaque 73, Renographin 60 and 73, Renographin 60 and 75, Amipaque, Isopaque Conray 80, Conray 420, Omnipaque.

Properties:

a. It is miscible with body fluids and saliva.
b. They have an iodine content ranging from 28–30 w/w and viscosity ranging from 2–10 centipoise.
c. These media are all hypertonic in comparision with plasma and saliva.

Advantages:

a. Their physical characteristics permit filling of the finer ducts system—less pain and discomfort.
b. They are rapidly removed from the tissues.

Disadvantages:

a. They have less degree of radiographic density and contrast.
b. It requires radiographs to be made as soon as possible after instillation of the medium.

Technique of Sialography

Sialography is routinely performed on either parotid or submandibular gland than the sublingual gland. Although the sublingual gland is difficult to infuse intentionally, it may be fortuitously opacified while infusing Wharton's duct to opacify the submandibular gland.

Important aspects and phases of a complete sialogram include an initial plain film examination of the gland at major draining duct, the retrograde injection of iodinated contrast medium and opacification of the ductal system and parenchyma, fluoroscopic spot films of the opacified ductal system and glandular parenchyma and post-evacuation films of the ductal system.

A survey (Scout) is usually made prior to the introduction of the contrast solution into the ductal system to aid in determining the correct exposure and patient positioning parameters. Radiopaque calculi may also be demonstrated, along with extraglandular and bone disease that may in fact be responsible for the clinical symptoms.

Techniques for Introducing the Contrast Media

A lacrimal probe (Bowman's or Liebreich's graduated lacrimal probe) is used to dilate the sphincter at the ductal orifice prior to passing a cannula (blunt needle or catheter) connected by extension tubing to a syringe containing contrast agent (Figs 5.1A and B).

There are three main techniques available for introducing the contrast medium into the ductal system.

Simple Injection Technique

Lipid soluble (e.g. ethiodol) or non-lipid soluble (e.g. sinographin) contrast solution is slowly introduced using gentle hand pressure until the patient experiences tightness or discomfort in the gland.

Advantages: of this technique is that it is simple and inexpensive.

Disadvantages:

- The arbitrary pressure which is applied may cause damage to the gland.
- Reliance on patient's responses may lead to under filling or overfilling of the gland.

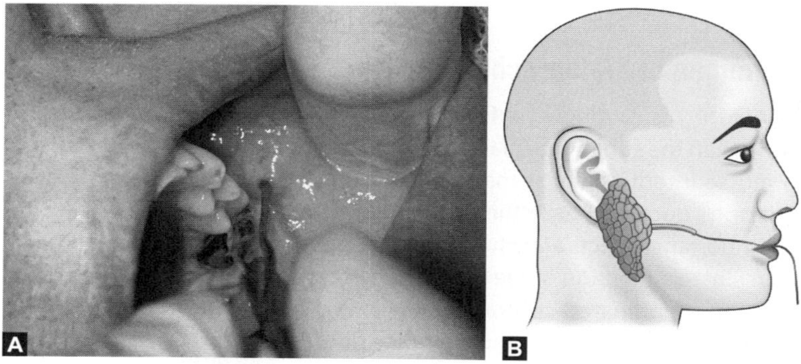

Figs 5.1A and B: (A) Insertion of cannula in salivary gland duct; (B) Contrast media is injected in salivary gland duct

Hydrostatic Technique

Aqueous contrast media is allowed to flow freely into the gland under the force of gravity until the patient experiences discomfort.

Advantages:

- The controlled introduction of contrast medium is less likely to cause damage or give an artifactual picture.
- It is simple and inexpensive.

Disadvantages:

a. Reliance on the patient's response.
b. Patients have to lie down during the procedure, so they need to be positioned in advance for the filling phase radiographs.

Continuous Infusion Pressure-monitored Technique

Using the aqueous contrast medium, a constant flow rate is adopted and the ductal pressure monitored throughout the procedure.

Advantages:

a. The controlled introduction of contrast media at known pressure is not likely to cause damage.
b. Does not cause overfilling of the gland.
c. Does not rely on the patients responses.

Disadvantages:

a. Complex equipment is required.
b. Time consuming.

Each of these techniques has its advocates, and with experience, each produces satisfactory results. The technique employed is therefore dependent on the operator and the facilities available.

PHASES OF SIALOGRAPHY

In evaluating any sialogram, it is important for the radiologist interpreting the study to observe, evaluate and comment on each phase and subphase in the final report. Direct observation allows the radiologist to observe the movement of contrast medium through the ductal system and obtain appropriate spot films that optimally show an abnormality that might not be evident or readily apparent on standard views, e.g. movement of small radiolucent stones or fistulae, as well as showing possible complications, for example, ductal rupture and/or extravasations that necessitate the immediate termination of the study.

Phases of sialography are as follows:
1. Ductal phase.
2. Acinar phase.
3. Post-evacuation phase.

The Ductal Phase

Of both the parotid and submandibular sialogram starts with the retrograde injection of the contrast medium and ends when the glandular parenchyma starts to become "hazy", reflecting the onset of acinar opacifications. The normal opacified parotid ductal system is often described as having a "leafless tree" appearance with a progressive gradual decrease in ductal caliber because branching of the various ducts occurs throughout the gland.

The image of the ductal system appears as "tree limbs" with no area of the gland devoid of ducts. With acinar filling the tree comes into "bloom" which is the typical appearance of the parenchymal opacification phase .

Visualization of duct(s) draining the accessory parotid gland(s) often occurs during the ductal phase. Appropriate spot films that should be routinely obtained following ductal opacifications include an anteroposterior, a puffed anteroposterior view of cheek, and a lateral view. Additional spot films that optimally show an abnormality or complication should also be obtained.

Anatomically and sialographically the submandibular or Wharton's duct can be divided into two distinct segments; a vertical or superficial segment below the level of the mylohyoid muscle, the deep segment which often unites with the sublingual or Bartholin's duct before entering the oral cavity. The normal, opacified submandibular ductal system often shows abrupt changes in ductal caliber as branching occurs; this is in marked contrast to orderly arborization seen in intraglandular parotid duct. Fluoroscopic spot films of the opacified submandibular duct obtained during ductal opacification should include films of the opacified, deep, horizontal portion of the primary duct, as well as an anteroposterior view and lateral oblique view of the completely opacified ductal system. An especially important area to visualize on the submandibular sialogram is the deep segment of the primary duct because the majority of submandibular sialoliths occur in this segment. In addition to the standard extraoral views, submentovertex view using intraoral films can be especially useful in showing pathology involving the deep segment of the submandibular duct.

The Acinar Phase

Starts with the completion of ductal opacification and ends when there is a generalized, increased density to the gland reflecting filling of glandular acini. In the pre-CT era, this phase was especially important in showing the possible presence of intraglandular masses. However, because nearly all sialograms are currently being performed to assess for ductal abnormalities, this phase is not as critical as it once was. Appropriate views for this phase of a sialogram include an anteroposterior and lateral view in the case of the parotid, and an anteroposterior and lateral oblique view in the case of the submandibular gland.

The Evacuation Phase

This is useful in assessing the secretory function of the gland, as well as accentuating any ductal pathology that might not have been readily apparent during other phases. The evacuation phase can be divided into two distinct subphases.

The first subphases lasts approximately 60 seconds and assess the unstimulated, spontaneous clearing of contrast from the gland. The second subphase assesses glandular clearing of intraductal and/or intraparenchymal contrast following stimulation with a sialogogue, e.g. lemon juice. This phase is performed only if there is incomplete spontaneous clearing of contrast during the first subphase. Both phases are performed under intermittent fluoroscopy. Nonclearing or incomplete clearing of a gland during either phase can be due to a sialolith and/or stricture, extraducatal or extravasated contrast, collection of contrast in abscess cavities, or an underlying physiologic abnormality.

Interpretation Requires

- A systematic approach
- A detailed knowledge of the radiographic appearances of normal salivary glands
- A detailed knowledge of the pathological conditions affecting the salivary glands.

Sialographic Appearances of the Normal Parotid Gland

- The main duct is of even diameter (1–2 mm wide) and should be filled completely and uniformly
- The duct structure within the gland branches regularly and tapers gradually toward the periphery of the gland, the so-called "tree in winter" appearance (Figs 5.2A and B).

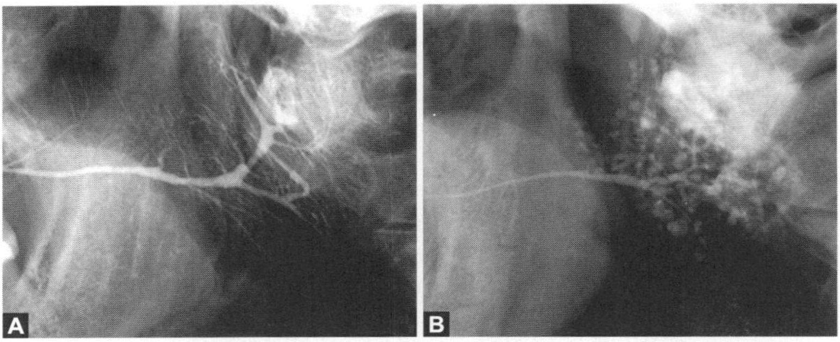

Figs 5.2A and B: (A) Normal sialographic appearance of parotid gland—"Tree in winter appearance"; (B) Normal sialographic appearance of submandibular gland "Bush in winter appearance"

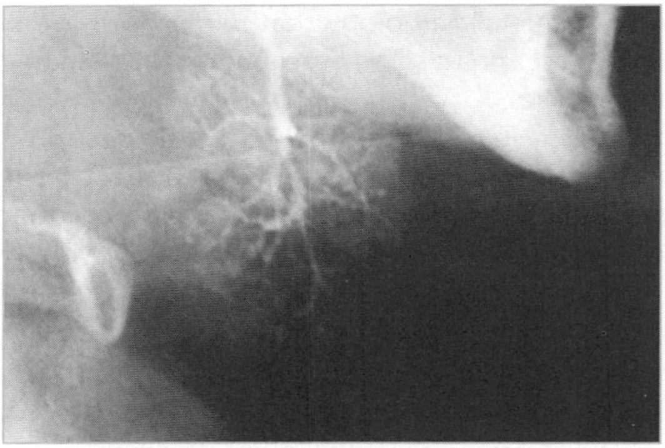

Fig. 5.3: Sialogram of normal submandibular gland

Sialography Appearance of the Normal Submandibular Gland

- The main duct is of even diameter (3–4 mm wide) and should be filled completely and uniformly.
- This gland is smaller than the parotid, but the overall appearance is similar with the branching duct structure tapering gradually toward the periphery, the so-called "bush in winter appearance" (Fig. 5.3).

Sialographic Appearance of Calculi

- Filling defects in the main duct
- Ductal dilatation caused by associated sialodochitis
- The emptying film usually shows contrast medium retained behind the stone (Figs 5.4 and 5.5).

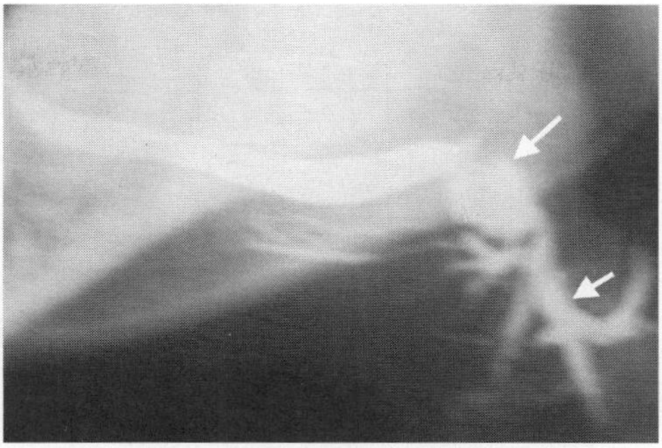

Fig. 5.4: Sialogram—left submandibular gland showing a large calculus within the gland "sausage—link" appearance

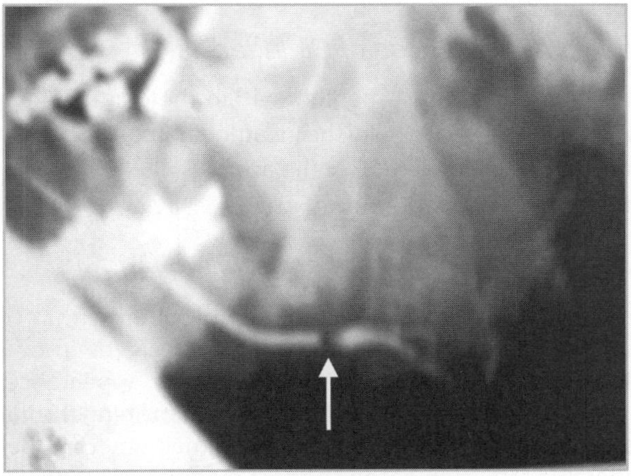

Fig. 5.5: Sialography—lateral view of submandibular gland demonstrating sialolith in the main duct

Sialographic Appearances of Sialodochitis (Ductal Inflammation/ Infection)

- Segment sacculation or dilatation and stricture of the main duct, the so-called "sausage link" appearance
- Associated calculi or ductal stenosis (Fig. 5.6).

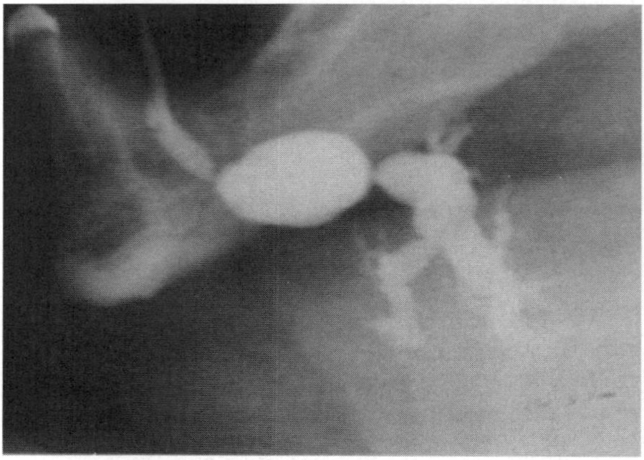

Fig. 5.6: Sialograph—lateral view of submandibular gland shows prominent intermittent stricture and dilation of main and secondary ducts

Sialographic Appearances of Sialadenitis

- Dots or blobs of contrast medium within the gland, an appearance known as sialectasis caused by the inflammation of the glandular tissue producing saccular dilatation of the acini.
- The main duct is usually normal (Fig. 5.7).

Sialographic Appearances in Sjögren's Syndrome

- Widespread dots or blobs of contrast medium within the gland, an appearance known as "punctate sialectasis" or "snowstorm" or "branchless fruit laden tree", or "cherry blossom" appearance.
- This is caused by a weakening of the epithelium lining the intercalated ducts, allowing the escape of the contrast medium from the ducts.
- Considerable retention of the contrast medium during the emptying phase.
- The main duct is usually normal (Fig. 5.8).

Sialographic Appearance of Intrinsic Tumors

- An area of under-filling within the gland, due to ductal compression by the tumor.
- Ductal displacement—the ducts adjacent to the tumor are usually stretched around it, an appearance known as "ball in hand".
- Retention of contrast medium in the displaced ducts during the emptying phase (Fig. 5.9).

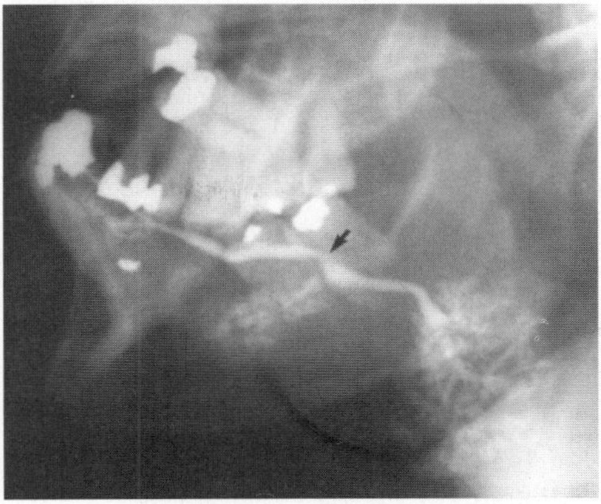

Fig. 5.7: Stricture on the middle part of the main duct and sialectasis in sublingual and submandibular gland (Chronic sialadenitis)

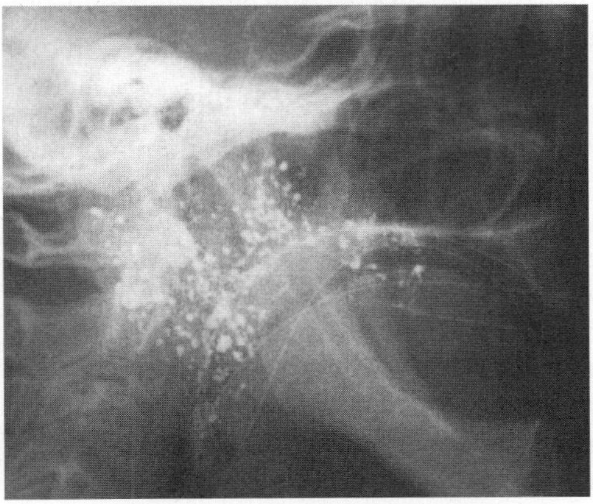

Fig. 5.8: Sjögren's syndrome—"snowstorm" appearance of punctate sialectasis

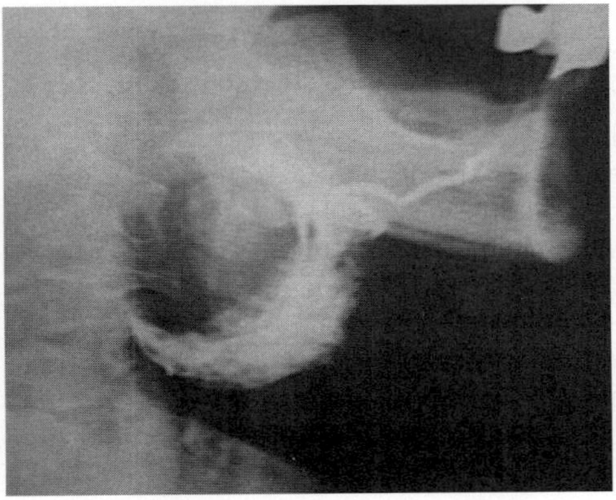

Fig. 5.9: "Ball in hand" appearance in pleomorphic adenoma in submandibular gland

Complications of Sialography

Usually, there are no complications from sialography. Overdistention of gland may cause temporary swelling and discomfort for a few hours to a few days. Extravasation of contrast media particularly oil soluble contrast may result in foreign body reaction. The iodide compounds used in sialography may rarely cause "lodine mumps". It is a bilateral enlargement of salivary glands following administration of iodied compounds. The mechanism of "lodine mumps" is unknown Kohiri suggested that a high concentration of iodide in the saliva causes inflammation of salivary gland and ductal mucosa. This in turn obstructs the excretion of saliva causing the gland to swell.

Study done by Nicholas A Drage, Jackie E Brown shows: sialography was performed in 92 patients. There was pain and swelling one hour after sialogram, the swelling returned to base line level after one day. A reduction in pain to below base line level was noted 2 days after sialography, which may suggest an unexpected benefit of sialography.

The use of iodinated contrast is contraindicated in patients with iodine allergy. The use of the gadolinium (gadopentate dimeglumine) as an alternate contrast agent is suggested by Williams MD, Moody AB et al.

A study was done by Wouter WI Kalk et al to evaluate the morbidity and acceptability of parotid sialography using oil based contrast media, conclusion is parotid sialography appears less invasive than it is often thought. It had a low morbidity rate and was well accepted by the patients. Twenty-four consecutive sialographic procedures were evaluated in terms of morbidity and the patient's acceptance of the procedure, assessed with a standardized questionnaire. Information was also obtained by recording relevant physical parameters during the procedure.

SIALOENDOSCOPY

Sialography is necessary to determine whether sialoendoscopy should be performed as a therapeutic procedure for the salivary obstructive disorders, especially for sialoliths. The endoscopic mechanical retrieval of sialoliths is both safe and efficacious. This is an excellent method for complete and certain removal of sialoliths with minimal damage to the surrounding tissue.

An article by Oded Nahlieli et al describes the use of endoscopy for diagnostic and surgical intervention in the major salivary gland of patients who have obstructive pathology. A total of 154 salivary glands suspected of having obstructive pathology. The ability to enter the ductal lumen was determined by measuring the duct, using the sialogram and the ultrasonogram.

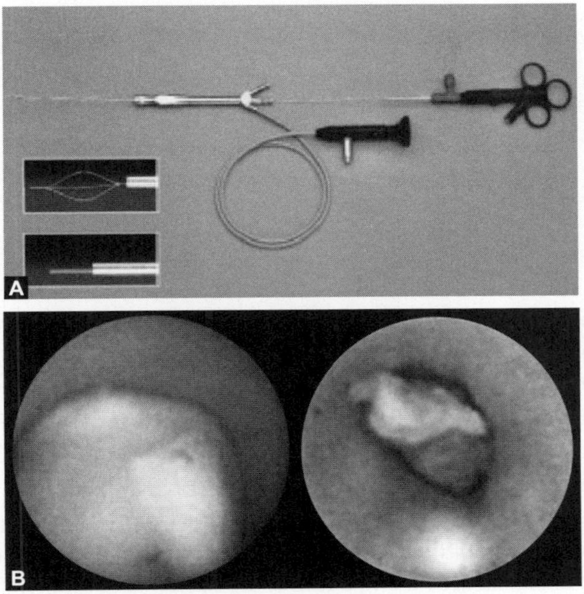

Figs 5.10A and B: (A) Endoscope used for dilatation of salivary ducts; (B) Endoscopic image of salivary duct

Sialography was used for mapping the ductal system, for possible variations and estimating potential inflation capability (Figs 5.10A and B).

Indications of Sialoendoscopy

1. Calculus removal that could not be performed by conventional methods.
2. Screening of the salivary ductal system for residual calculi after sialolithotomy.
3. Positive evidence of ductal dilatation or stenosis on the sialogram or ultrasound examination.
4. Recurrent episodes of major salivary gland swellings without known cause.

Sialoendoscopy is minimally invasive technique which works fine in many obstructive disorders of salivary glands.

ANGIOGRAPHY

Angiography, a radiographic procedure carried out by injecting radiopaque dye into vessels and making radiographs. When the dye is located in the vasculature, it is useful for demonstrating the size and extent of a vascular tumor of the jaw. It displays an abnormal collection of vessels located in the suspected area, with many vessles feeding and draining the lesion. Angiography demonstrates the nature of the vascular derangement, its relationship to the bone defect, and associated abnormal arterial and venous vasculature.

Angiography includes arteriography and phlebography.

Arteriography is important in study of salivary tumors because it not only defines the vasculature of tumor but also delineates the origin of vasculalure of tumor. Delineation of the blood supply can aid the surgeon in pre-operative evaluation of surgical procedure being planned for patient. The arteriogram of tumor shows displacement of rigid and streched vessels surrounding the tumor mass, abnormal vascularity with persistent distortion and pooling of contrast media and early venous return.

Contrast Media in Arteriography

Arteriography ideally require a medium that gives good contrast, possess low viscosity (for rapidity of injection) and is nontoxic. The contrast media that have universal use for angiography are sodium and methylglucamine diatrizoate, metrizoate, Iohexol, Iopamidol and Ioxaglate. Gadodiamide and ultrasmall superparamagnetic iron oxide (SPIO) can also be used for imaging the vascular system.

The normal external carotid artery can be opacified by 3–10 mL of contrast medium. Low osmolarity and non tonic contrast media are used in phlebography or venography where it can be injected by either direct puncture of the vein or indirectly by injecting the medium into the arterial system and imaging the venous return. Contrast medium can also be injected intraosseously and the venous drainage imaged.

6 Arthrography

On conventional radiograph the image is formed as a result of differential attenuation of an X-ray beam by the structures through which the X-ray pass. Structures that lack sufficient density to attenuate the beam do not appear on the radiograph. If the density of a structure of interest is too low to be visualized on an X-ray image or if the subject contrast is too low to meet specific diagnostic need, the contrast and density can be improved artificially.

Artificial contrast is produced in a variety of ways. Material with high coefficient of absorption can be placed in or around the structure of interest. Radiographically invisible structures can be visualized by using artificially induced contrast. Artificially induced contrasts are also helpful in allowing density to evaluate structures that would otherwise be radiographically invisible. Opaque matter is incorporated into otherwise radiolucent materials.

DEFINITION

The introduction of opaque fluid into joint spaces followed by X-ray examination of the joint. This is commonly used to examine the anatomy of large joints, particularly the knee and shoulder. But it is also useful for evaluation of temporomandibular joint (TMJ) diseases. This technique is called as arthrography.

CONTRAST AGENT

Modern contrast agent used in the evaluation of biologic structures and function are compound of iodine. These agents must be evaluated in terms of their toxicity, viscosity and mode of excretion.

In general, most contrast agents can be divided into two major categories:

a. Water soluble
b. Fat soluble

Water soluble materials are often intended for intravenous injection, whereas fat soluble contrast agents are most commonly used to outline other, non-vascular existing bony cavities. Fat soluble agents generally provide more contrast than their water soluble counter parts.

Water soluble materials are preferred in the examination of joint. They provide enough contrast to define extra-articular structures and they have the advantages of being dissipated quickly.

RATIONALE

The basic objective of arthrography is to opacify the joint synovial spaces so that subsequent radiograph may provide images of the articular disk and its attachment (Fig. 6.1).

The procedure is performed by inserting, needle and catheter under fluoroscopic guidance, into the joint space and injecting water soluble contrast medium (dye). Radiographs are taken in various stages of joint function. The articular disk and its attachments are seen as radiolucent

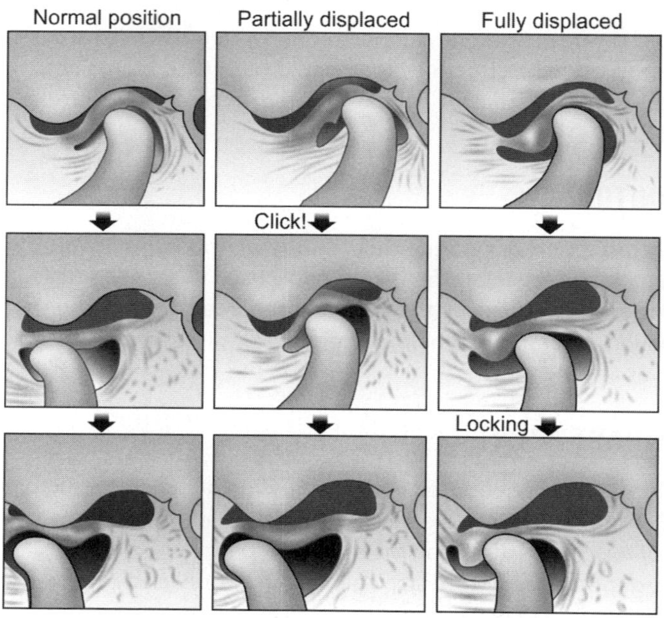

Fig. 6.1: Position and movement of the disk during jaw opening. Normal position (left) mildly anteriorly displaced, with reduction (in middle). Severely displaced anteriorly, without reduction (right)

areas projecting between pools of opaque contrast medium. Identifying the precise position and morphology structure of these soft tissues is the main goal of any arthrographic procedure.

Temporomandibular joint arthrography is presently useful diagnostically when the clinician is in doubt as to whether derangement (including displacement, perforation or deformation) of the articular disk or its posterior attachment is present. The procedure can provide critical diagnostic information regarding the articular disk that is obtainable only by direct surgical inspection. Specifically such information includes the precise position of disk relative to the condyle, the morphological structure of the disk and the presence of tear of disk, perforation or adhesion in the disk or posterior attachment (Fig. 6.2).

INDICATIONS

1. One purpose of TMJ arthrography is to confirm the clinical diagnosis.
2. Surgeon may elect to obtain an arthrogram to have information about the soft tissue.
3. When surgeon is not certain that patient has internal derangement arthrogram is indicated.
4. To obtained specific information about disk position and morphology.
5. To document the diagnosis and extent of derangement.

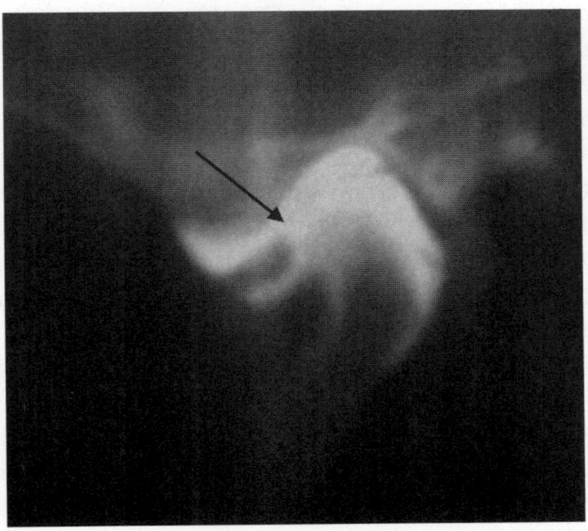

Fig. 6.2: A single contrast arthrogram showing perforation immediately posterior to a deformed disk

CONTRAINDICATIONS

1. Should be performed with caution in patient who has history of reaction to contrast medium.
2. Bleeding disorders and anticoagulation medications are relative contraindications.
3. Should not be performed in presence of localized skin infection because of risk of introducing infection to joint.
4. Special risks exist in patient with impaired renal function.
5. It is contraindicated in patient undergoing thyroid function test.

COMPLICATIONS

1. Accidental introduction of contrast material into brain through the roof of the glenoid fossa may produce convulsions and possible fatal reaction.
2. Contrast agents can cause shock, local allergic reaction and inflammatory condition.

TECHNIQUE

Arthrography must be performed as a sterile procedure under fluoroscopic observation. Although it is not essential, premedication of patient is desirable. Administration of 20–40 mg of diazepam by mouth approximately 40 minutes before the examination is usually sufficient. Local anesthesia is achieved with up to 4 mL of 1% lidocaine infiltrated around the area of the joint.

The process of entering the upper and lower joint spaces for the infusion of radiographic contrast medium may be accomplished with either needles or angiocatheters. The use of angiocatheters for this purpose was introduced by Wilkes. The angiocatheter plastic tube is flexible and has blunt tip; these factors reduce the danger of laceration of the joint soft tissues. Having the flexibility to adjust contrast volumes during an examination is another practical reason to use angiocatheter as indwelling tubes.

Separate injections of the contrast agents (renografin 60 or hypaque 60) are required to delineate the upper and lower joint compartments. With the patient under fluoroscopic observation and with the mouth partially open, 0.3–0.5 mL of water soluble radiographic contrast medium is injected into lower joint space. The posterior recess of the lower space should be opacify. The injected contrast medium should be confined to distinct space. When the mouth is closed, most the contrast medium will transfer to the anterior recess. If any of the contrast medium fills the upper joint space as well, a perforation in the disk (or the posterior attachment) is denoted, the injection continued until optimal feeling is seen fluoroscopically.

The examiner is cautioned to avoid over injecting as this may damage the capsule or internal tissues and cause considerable diskomfort to the patient when the local anesthesia resolves.

The upper space is similarly injected. The upper space will accommodate slightly more contrast medium than the lower space.

Radiography

Radiography of the opacified joint spaces must be performed as soon as possible after filling it with contrast medium, preferably within 5 minutes sooner the radiographs are produced, better the images of the joint spaces. Tomography should be used to produce nondistorted images through the crucial lateral and central aspects of the joint.

Projections are routinely made with the jaws closed and at various degrees of opening. In cases that involve a clicking joint, one of the several open jaw projections are made just as the patient thinks that click is imminent (Figs 6.3A and B).

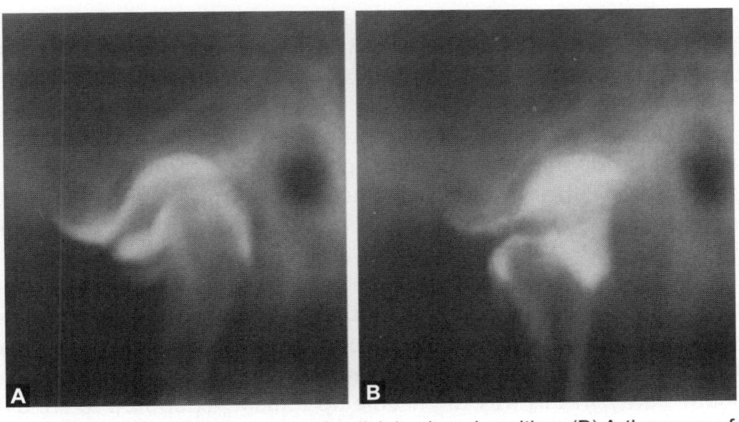

Figs 6.3A and B: (A) Arthrogram of a disk in closed position; (B) Arthrogram of a disk in open position

POSTOPERATIVE COURSE

After the radiography phase of the arthrographic examination, the angicoatheters are pulled, the skin puncture site is bandaged and cold pack is applied to the area. The contrast medium injected into the joint will be gradually absorbed by the synovium and carried through the bloodstream to the kidneys, where its removal from the body is initiated.

Two short term effects after arthrography are sometime observed. First, the patient may noticed an altered dental occlusion caused by the fluid injection into joint spaces. Second patient should expect mild-to-moderate diskomfort in the region of TMJ after local anesthesia resolves. The analgesics of moderate strength should be prescribed.

DOUBLE CONTRAST ARTHROTOMOGRAPHY

Single contrast arthrography is the filling of the joint compartment with radiopaque contrast medium before radiography. The single contrast technique is usually combined with tomography, improving the radiographic representation of the joint.

In double contrast arthrography, the articular surfaces are coated by radiopaque medium and joint compartment is expanded by air. The information from double contrast arthrography has been consider to be superior to that result from single contrast arthrography.

TECHNIQUE

Patient is transfer to fluoroscopic unit and placed in supine position. Then the head is positioned on image intensifier and turned about 80° toward the side not be examined. The X-ray tube which is placed superiorly is tilted 5° to 10° caudally against the vertical plane. In this way, lateral oblique transcranial projection of TMJ is obtained, projection is controlled by fluoroscopic and adjusted to achieve optical image of the joint. This is done under local anesthesia which is obtained by infiltration of about 0.8 mL of lidocaine HCL 2% with epinephrine 1:80000 into the tissues posterior to the condyle and 0.5 mL inferior to the articular tubercle.

The lower compartment is cannulated first by insertion of a cannula (1.1 × 32) posterior to the condyle. With patients mouth closed cannula is directed against posterior surface of condyle and bone contact is reached. The position is fluoroscopically checked. Then the patient is asked to open mouth slowly. In this way the needle tip remain juxtaposed to condyle during movement. The inner needle is withdrawn and catheter is medially advanced into posterior recess of the lower compartment.

Then the upper joint compartment is cannulated with patient mouth closed. The level of cannula is oriented superioanteriorly. The cannula is inserted about 10 mm for lower compartment and directed against posterior slope of articular tubercle. As bone contact is obtained the position is fluoroscopically checked. If the position is correct the inner needle is withdrawn and catheter is medially advanced into upper compartment.

After placement of catheter about 0.2–0.3 mL contrast agent is injected into lower and upper compartment respectively via extension tubes under fluoroscopic observation.

After injection into lower compartment single exposure is made to document the location of contrast medium. After successful cannulation the contrast medium in lower compartment should flow freely around the condyle and in the upper compartment along the articular tubercle. During injection contrast medium should enter the joint without resistance.

The tips of catheter are left in the joint compartment and outer part of catheter is fixed to the skin with tape. Then the patient is transferred to tomographic unit and immobilized with 2 head, in the cephalostat in original position. With mouth of patient at maximum opening another 0.3–0.5 mL contrast agent is injected into lower compartment and tomography is performed.

While the mouth is closed, contrast medium is allowed to reflux in order to avoid overexpansion and rupture of compartment. Arthrotomography is then performed in the intercuspal position. With the aid of catheter in the joint compartment most of iodine contrast medium is aspirated. Then by using glass syringe with low friction and another pair of extention tubes, air is injected into both the compartment simultaneously until an elastic resistance is experienced.

Amount of air injected ranges from 0.2–0.6 mL and 0.1–0.4 mL for upper and lower compartment. Care is to be taken that double contrast arthrograms are obtained at maximum mouth opening and in intercuspal position.

Advantages of Double Contrast Arthrography

1. Double contrast arthrotomography of TMJ is able to demonstrate the position and configuration of the disk with its anterior and posterior attachment.
2. In single contrast medium the entire joint compartments are filled with highly radiopaque contrast medium, under this circumstances contrast material located outside tomographic plane give rise to radiopaque

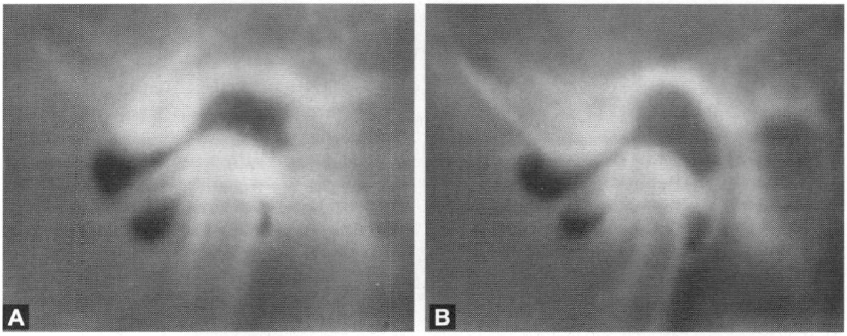

Figs 6.4A and B: (A) Double contrast arthrography (Joint space appears radiolucent and the disk is radiopaque): The disk is displaced anterior to the condylar head in the closed position; (B) Remains displaced in the open position

pseudo image, this impairs the radiographic representation of anatomic structures, because air in double contrast arthrography, constituted the major portion of contrast material, this undesirable effect is largely avoided (Figs 6.4A and B).

Normal TMJ Arthrogram

The articular disk is seen as the biconcave water interposed between the bony articulating surfaces. In an actual arthrogram the posterior aspect of the disk merges imperceptibly with posterior attachment, both of which normally occupy much of joint space above condylar head. The clear areas in the drawing between the bony surfaces are the upper and lower joints spaces. Each space in divided into an anterior and posterior recess. The upper and lower joints spaces do not communicate with each other. The articulating surface of the condyle is normally positioned against the under surface of the thin central portion of the disk, the bony convexity fitting neatly into the concavity of the disk of particular diagnostic importance is the observation that the relationship of the condyle to the think portion of the disk is constant throughout the opening and closing sequences of joint movement. There is a smooth, harmonious relationship between these two joint structures in movements.

With the teeth in occlusion, the anterior recess of the upper and lower joint compartments are relatively distended with contrast medium. As the condyle begins to translate during jaw opening, a portion of contrast medium is hydraulically forced form the anterior the posterior recess. As the condyle continues forward, the posterior recesses increasingly assumed characteristic shapes. The upper posterior recess resembled the top half of round white disk; the lower posterior recess assumes a shape similar to halve of heart. At full opening, the anterior recesses are virtually obliterated as contrast medium extrudes to the posterior joint recesses.

Anterior Displacement of Disk with Reduction

Arthography may be performed in cases in which an audible click or a popping sensation is associated with occasional painful limitation of opening. Arthrography can often demonstrated the mechanics of click, which tend to occur in reciprocal manner as the condyle translates anteriorly and posteriorly.

The closed mouth arthrograms image of clicking joint will typically show the disk situated, not in a normal anterosuperior relationship to the codyle but in anterior position. The condylar articulating surface is positioned just posterior to thick band of the disk. The lower anterior recess is elongated and more horizontal when compared with normal arthrograms. As the jaw begin to open and condyle moves toward, the disk is carried forward by shearing force of the condyle. At the same point during condyle translation, the posterior band of the disk recoils over condylar articulating surface and in doing so established a normal disk condyle relationship. This posterior recall of the disk occurs quickly. After the typical recoil movement, a normal and harmonious relationship is achieved between disk and condyle for the reminder of the opening the sequence. When the mouth is closed, the relationship of the disk and condyle remains normal until clicking point is reached here upon the disk is again displayed forward.

Anterior Displacement of the Disk without Reduction

As seen both clinically and arthrographically, TMJ that manifested a closed lock has a more advanced abnormality than does the TMJ that has reciprocal click or pop during opening closing movements. With the teeth in occlusion, the disk is positioned anterior to the articulating surface of condyle head, even more so than in the clicking situation. The condyle itself is slightly retruded in the joint, direct reflection of anterior displacement of the disk. As the condyle goes through early and mid-range translation, it picks up the posterior rim of the disk and forces it further forward. At no point during the anterior movement of condyle does, the disk spontaneously recoil posteriorly over condylar head. No reduction of the displacement of the disk occurs. In fact, at maximal jaw opening, the disk physically blocks the condyle from achieving a normal excursion. As the final feature, disk is obtained progressively deformed during such as opening lock sequence.

The cause of deformation is the compressive force generated by the condyle as the latter is pulled forward by muscle action.

If both the joint spaces opacify after infusion of contrast medium into only one space, it may be predicted with near certainly that pathologic perforation of the disk or the posterior attachment exists. In such cases, the contrast medium flows through the perforation and into noninjected joint space.

7 Arthroscopy

Arthroscopy is valuable adjunctive imaging technique for the temporomandibular joint (TMJ). Unlike other imaging modalities arthroscopy lessens joint pain and improves disk dynamics. Arthroscopy has bridged the gap between nonsurgical temporomadibular joint surgery and the open joint surgery (arthrotomy). It allows direct visualization providing information that until recently was available only by arthrotomy.

Ohinishi was the first to describe the application of arthroscopy to the TMJ . He along with Murakami and Kino defined the terminology, pathology and anatomy of TMJ arthroscopy. In vivo arthroscopic TMJ research in United States was reported first by Hilsa Beck, Kaskin and by Williams.

The development of smaller arthroscope and surgical proficiency provided data for studies that confirmed the reliability of arthroscopy. Using sweeping and lavage of superior joint compartment, over 90% of patient with persistently anteriorly displaced disk experienced reduced pain and increased function, even though disk recapture was not present postoperatively (Figs 7.1A and B).

Moses and Pocker suggest that the success of arthroscopy may be attributed to:

1. Removal of inflammatory substance by lavage (hypothesizing that some of these substance were pain transmitter).

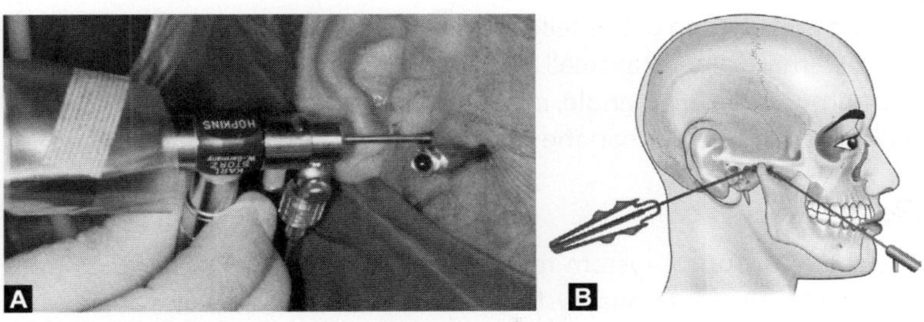

Figs 7.1A and B: (A) Extraoral position and site of arthroscope insertion in TMJ space; (B) Position and site of arthroscope insertion in TMJ space

2. Increased disk mobility.
3. Reduced adverse wading of supporting joint structure.
4. Reduction of synovial inflammation as a possible cause of muscle strain and fatigue.

INSTRUMENTATION

Arthroscope

The arthroscopy is essentially cylinders that conduct light into cavity and transmits an image back to the eye. Several small joint arthroscopic systems are currently available, e.g. the temporomandibular joint. The optical principle of each telescopic system fall into one of the three categories: traditional lens system, selfoscope lens system and rod lens system. The traditional lens system and rod lens system are example of rigid endoscopy, in which the transmitting mechanism is a series of lenses and the illuminating mechanism is a fiber bundle. The selfoscope system is somewhere between rigid endoscopy and fiber optic endoscopy.

Traditional Lens System

The traditional optical system consists of long narrow tube with series of small glass relay and field lenses assembled at specific intervals with intervening air spaces. To reduce the effect of stray light on the contrast of the final image, the inner surface of the tube is corrugated or rifled.

Selfoscope Lens System

The selfoscope system consists of a long, narrow tube containing a single image transmitting fiber and multiple incoherent illuminating fibers. The transmitting fiber, diameter 0.5–1.0 mm is specially treated to improve its refractive index.

The engineering of the selfoscope system allows fabrication of system with external diameter as small as 1.7 mm. However, limitation in the degree of brightness, viewing angle, color, resolution and contrast of selfoscope make it less desirable than the rod lens system.

Rod Lens System

The rod lens optical system reverses the function of air and glass from that used in the traditional system. Air lenses and glass spaces are used to improve light transmission. The capacity of the telescope to transmit light is directly proportional to the square of refractive index of relay lenses. The glass spaces of rod lens system have an index of approximately 1.5–1.6. This index compare favorably to that of air (N = 100).

The rod lens system has several advantages over the other system. They are as follows:

a. A brighter image results from decreased light absorption.
b. The diagnostic capability is improved owing to wider viewing angle.
c. The rod lens system provides improved contrast, color reproduction and resolution.

Solid Instrument

The basic instrument for penetration and exploration of the joint are the same for each arthroscopic system. These instrument are categorized as capsule penetration instrument, hand held surgical instrument and motorized surgical instrument.

Capsule Penetration Instrument

For capsule penetration, each system contains three principle components: external sheath, sharp trocar (obturator) and blunt trocar. Small differences in design exist as length of instruments and the type of locking mechanism. External sheaths, blunt trocars and sharp trocar of varying diameters and length are available to accommodate hand and motor instruments or to act as an outflow port when a two-part system is used.

Hand Held Instrument

A probe is an effective tool in both diagnostic and operative arthroscopy. By virtue of the dull hook at its distal end, the probe may be used to practice triangulation, retract the retrodiscal tissue and check the consistency of remodeled retrodiskal tissue and disk.

The pediatric urethrotome may be adopted for operative arthroscopy. This instrument can be used as a single instrument for diagnostic and operative arthroscopy. A 0-degree telescope is mounted in tandem to a cutting instrument. The external sheath can thus accommodate the telescope, cutting instrument and irrigant. Rosette, straight sickle and retrograde knives are available.

A trigger allows the operator to control the movement of knife in and out of external sheath. The external sheath is elliptical and measures 4 mm in maximum diameter. This instrument may be useful in cutting diseased tissue.

Scissor and punch forceps with long working arms may be introduced through the external sheath of second part. A variety of instrument designs permit the retrieval of foreign bodies, removal of small pieces of tissue and incision of adhesion.

A variety of arthroscopic knives with different configuration may be used to incise tissue. These instruments have proven to be most effective in cutting remodeled retrodiskal tissue. They pass readily through the short external sheath of second part. Unfortunately, they need to be replaced frequently because they dull quickly, and various blade configuration makes resharpening difficult red rubber or silicone tubing may be used to cover the edges.

A malleable tension arm is available to assist in holding the telescope during operative arthroscopy. The arm attached to the side of operating table. The tension of arm may be adjusted so that it can carry the telescope with the weight video camera or articulated arm.

Motorized Instrument

The shaver consist of a hollow, distally fenestrated sheath containing a rotating cylindrical cutting instrument that can rotate within the hallow sheath. The cutting instruments are driven by motor, controlled by foot pedal. Cable driven and battery-powered models, as well as shavers containing power components, are available. Each type of shaver has its restriction with regard to sterilization.

The efficiency of the cutting instrument depend on several factor, including the strength of the motor, the proximity of the cutting instrument to the edge of the fenestration in the outer sheath and diameter of the lumen of sheath. The cutting instrument dull rapidly. The handle of the shaver has an attachment for suction that the arthroscopist may opt to apply while cutting.

ILLUMINATIONS

Several types of light sources are available. Xenon light provides brighter image with better color rendition then halogen light lamp output is adjustable. A series of adapter are sold to enable light cables of one manufacturer to mater the light source of another.

Fibers light cables are used for illumination only. They are composed of incoherent fiber bundles. Each cable contains multiple fiberglass threads that conduct light from the light source through the telescope and into the articular cavity. Each fiber has a diameter of about 25u (maicrone) and is composed of high-quality optical glass. A high refractive index core transmits; light and low refractive index cladding provide internal reflection for optimum conservation of light. Light may be internally reflected more than 15,000 times per meter in fiberglass light guide without cladding. Contamination of surface of the fiber would cause significant loss of light. Amount of light interning the joint cavity cannot be increased beyond the optimum light conducting efficiency of the finite number of fibers in telescope. Fluid light cables are also available. These cable conduct light through fluid medium. Photographic image will appear brighter. These cables are less flexible and the operator may initially find their stiffness difficult to manage.

PHOTOGRAPHY IN ARTHROSCOPY

The need for good documentation of arthroscopic procedure arose because of the widespread acceptance of diagnostic and surgical arthroscopy by the orthopedic community.

Whether the operators regard himself primarily as diagnostic arthroscopist or surgical the photographic record is of value. An accurate photographic record provides some degree of medicolegal protection. Videotape and slide material are excellent teaching aids and may be used in publication. Historically, the advancement and eventual adaptation of the endoscopic technique as an established orthopedic procedure was based on the development of sophisticated photographic method. For still photography following equipment is recommended.

1. Rod lenses telescope.
2. 35 mm single lens-reflex camera adaptable to the arthroscopy.
3. Ektachromo 400ASA for diapositives and kadacolor 400 ASA for prints.
4. A xenon light source, through a 150 watt halogen light source is acceptable.
5. Light source capable of regulating flash diskharge typically with TTL cable connecting the camera to the light source.
6. Lens with focal length of 60–130 mm—optical photograph have been obtained with magnification of 90 to 110 times.
7. Tri or stabilizing arm for camera.
8. Optional accessories include data back system and motor drive.

For video photography the following additional equipment is recommended.

1. Light weigh video camera.
2. Video recorder preferably a ¾ inch videotape recorder should be employed to permit optimal image resolution.

Advantages

1. Minimum histological changes after arthroscopic joint examination and lavage.
2. By maintaining the synovial cell the joint are enable to replenish and repair intracapsular structure, there by diminishing postoperative morbidity.
3. The improved visualization of joint structures that can be recorded on video tape and retrieved for documentation and future reference add to the superiority of arthroscopy.
4. Procedure can be accomplished in 10–30 minutes in which diagnosis and lavage were completed through small incision or puncture that did not always require suturing.
5. Jaw mobilization is immediate after arthroscopy with full range of motion resume within 3 days.
6. Cost of arthrography is lower than arthrotomy.
7. Use to confirm the position of articular disk before proceeding to orthodontic therapy and disk position was correlated with final tooth positioning.

Disadvantages

1. It is still invasive procedure although much less than arthrotomy.
2. Special training and equipment needed continue to limit its wide acceptance.
3. Learning curve for arthroscopy is believed to be substantially higher than arthrotomy.
4. Complications are potentially more serious such as middle ear perforation.
5. Arthroscopy does not permit the meticulous manipulation and suturing of malposition disk.

Arthroscopy Relative to Other Imaging Techniques

1. Arthroscopy should be used an adjunctive technique for visualizing the TMJ.
2. Arthroscopy provides clear visual demonstration of dynamic soft tissue anatomy as does video arthrography but can also detect synovitis and arthritis.
3. Arthrography provides better detail of condyles dynamics but perforation can be localized more precisely with arthroscopy.

4. CT appears to be less effective than arthroscopy and arthrography in demonstrating the size and shape of articular disk.
5. Arthrography will yield the best information about disk dynamics and arthroscopy the best information about disk integrity (Figs 7.2A and B).

TECHNIQUE OF ARTHROSCOPY

Arthroscopy is usually performed on an outpatient basis but under general anesthesia through nasoendotracheal intubation.The patient is prepared for preauricular approach and the surgical field is sterilized. The patient's mouth is draped with sterile drapes to allow surgeon's assistant to manipulate the mandible.

Arthroscope should be inserted slightly anterior to tragus of ear in line with lateral canthus of the eye. A 20 gauge needle attached to 10 mL syringe filled with normal saline is inserted into glenoid fossa from a point near tragus of ear and is directed anteriorly, superiorly and medially. Once the glenoid fossa is entered 3–5 mL of normal saline is injected to expand superior joint space, then after needle is removed a 2–4 mL vertical entry by incision is made anterior to tragus. A sharp trocar is placed through arthroscopic cannula and inserted in the same pathway as the needle that carried the normal saline. After lateral capsule is pierced with trocar, care is taken not to insert it further to avoid disruption of joint relationship, then an uniflow efflux needle is directed 5 mm anterior to arthroscopic cannula and lavaging the joint with normal saline confirms location. Heparinized lactated ringers may be used for joint irrigation and distention. The irrigation solution provide for expansion of the superior joint space so that examination and repair procedure can be accomplished more easily.

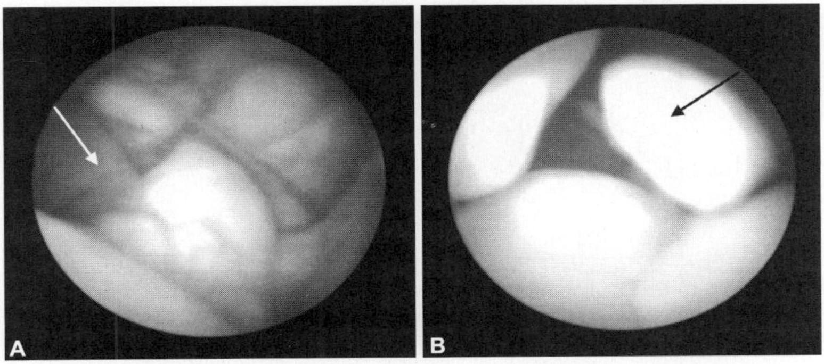

Figs 7.2A and B: Arthrographic image showing disk integrity

Ti is also used to remove debris and provide clear field of view and it also reduced the probability of intracapsular sepsis. A 0-degree wide angle 10 or 15-degree arthroscope is selected for diagnostic phase of procedure (Figs 7.3A to C).

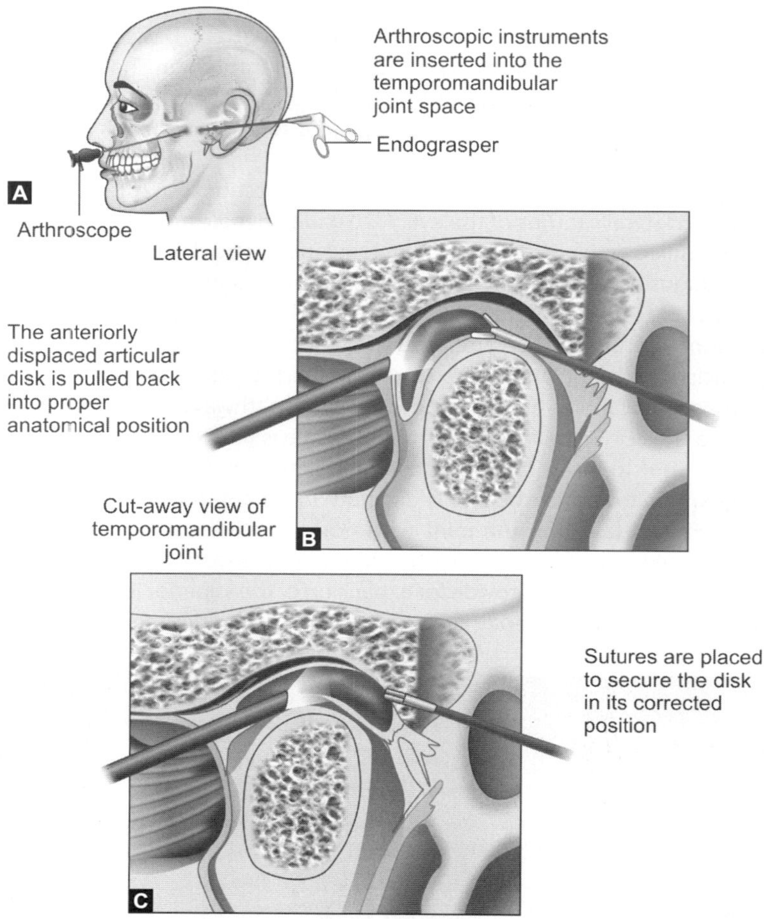

Figs 7.3A to C: Position of arthroscope in TMJ and relation between hard and soft tissue component of TMJ

The arthroscope is attached to fiberoptic light source that is coupled to video camera. A TV monitor is used for viewing that enlarged the field of view compare to viewing directing into lens of arthroscope. The fiberoptic bundles in the arthroscope illuminate the joint cavity and procedure is documented on videotape. Examination begins in the posterior joint recess by noting the integrity of the retrodiskal tissue. Ti is proceeded by noting the position of the disk and inclination of articular eminence.

Care is taken not to disrupt the fibrocartilage, covering the articular eminence so that adhesion or surface erosion can be documented, then manipulate the mandible to note the relationship of the articular disk to mandibular condyle, then proceed to the anteriosuperior recess which is often restricted due to lateral ligament and due to which covering of articular eminence is formed. Entrance to anterior recess is best gained either laterally or medially with the jaw in semi-closed position.

After examination joint is thoroughly lavaged and incision is closed with line suture. Corticosteroids are injected into capsule in cases with inflammatory or degenerative disease. Intraoral occlusal splint are inserted immediately after examination. Arthroscopic surgery done after joint examination except in cases where restrictive fibrosis prevents initial viewing. 30-degree arthroscope is preferred for panoramic viewing and for visualization of working instrument.

COMPLICATIONS

1. Extravasation of irrigation fluid into surrounding tissue occurs with over jealous irrigation.
2. Seventh cranial nerve damage.
3. Middle ear damage.
4. Blood vessel lysis.
5. Perforation of middle cranial fossa.
6. Breakage of instrument.

8 Nuclear Medicine

Nuclear medicine is a medical specialty uses safe, painless and cost-effective technique both to image the body and treat disease. It is unique in that it documents organ function, structure and quantitation. In contrast to diagnostic radiology, this is based upon anatomy by using very small amount of radioactive material. These procedures often identify abnormalities very early in the progression of a disease long before some medical problems are apparent with other diagnostic tests.

Nuclear medicine imaging technique is based on the principle of affinity of certain radioactive compound for particular target tissue. When these agents injected or swallowed by the patients concentrated in target tissue. It is very difficult to look inside the human body, but nuclear medicine imaging techniques give another way to look inside the human body with the help of radioactive elements. The techniques combine the use of computers, detectors, and substances.

These techniques include:

1. Positron emission tomography (PET)
2. Single photon emission computed tomography (SPECT)
3. Cardiovascular imaging
4. Bone scanning
5. Salivary gland scanning

Nuclear medicine technique can be used both for the therapeutic and diagnostic imaging. Radionuclides which emit β^- particles have great potential in the field of radionuclide therapy, while B^+ emitters provide the basis for positron emission tomography (PET).

For the purpose of therapy it is essential to have carrier-free isotopes, and with the exception of ^{33}P, ^{89}Sr, ^{90}Y, ^{125}I and ^{130}I, the β emitters of therapeutic interest are not commercially available. Therapeutic effects depend critically on the specific activity.

In imaging fast growing soft tissue gallium is commonly used in the form of 78 hours ^{67}Ga. The physical and biological half-lives and the γ-ray emitted are suitable for imaging.

One can commercially produce other Ga nuclides which either reduce the radiation dose to the patient during diagnosis or deliver increased dose to a tumor during treatment.

A number of isotope/radionuclide used in nuclear medicine for therapeutic and imaging purpose include:

Iodine-131

Iodine-131 is the most important and most commonly used, unsealed radionuclide for imaging. It decays by emission of β particle with a physical half-life of 8.1 days. Iodine is concentrated in the thyroid gland and this allows us to deliver a high radiation dose to the gland and a low dose to the rest of the body.

Phosphorus-32

Phosphorus-132 comes close to being the ideal unsealed therapeutic radionuclide. It is a pure β particle emitter with a physical half-life of 14.3 days. It is normally administered intravenously as sterile sodium phosphate, and is used in the treatment of polycythemia.

Yttrium-90

Yttrium-90 is also a pure β emitter with a physical half-life of 64.2 hours. An injection of a sterile suspension of colloidal yttrium silicate is given for a variety of disease states.

Strontium-89

Strontium-89, decay by β particle emission with a physical half-life of 50.5 days. From dental point of interest areas where the diagnostic isotopes are utilized, included head and neck tumor, salivary gland disease and various metabolic and infectious processes of the head and neck region.

Procedure

With the help of special gamma cameras, nuclear medicine studies where first done in 1950s. Nuclear medicine studies require the introduction of very low-level radioactive chemicals into the body. This "radionuclide" is distributed in the body based on the chemical composition of the molecules to which the radioactive atoms are attached. The intensity of the radiation source in nuclear medicine is much less then that in X-ray imaging (Fig. 8.1).

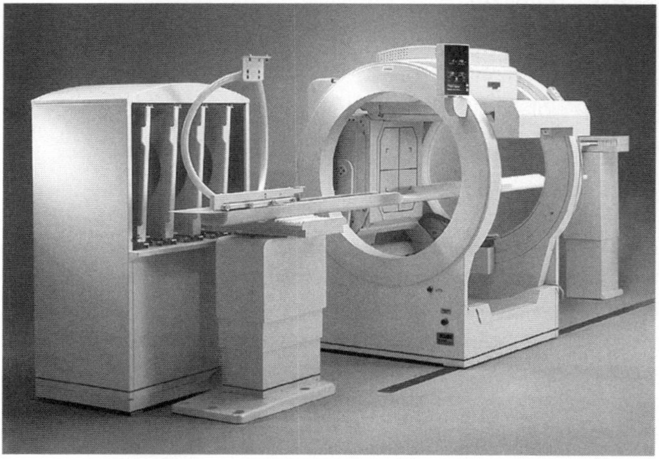

Fig. 8.1: Nuclear medicine machine spect system—gamma camera

Information is visualized using a gamma camera that contains a large crystal of sodium iodide, usually about 15 inches in diameter and 3/8" thick. This converts the γ-rays into the same way that the screen doses in X-ray imaging. Because the radiation intensity is so small the crystal has to be very thick. The individual light flashes from each γ-rays are detected by an array of very sensitive photomultiplier tubes mounted behind the crystal. The tube closest to where the γ-rays created the light flash in the crystal will detect the most light. The exact position of the source of the light will be determined from the relative amount of the light reaching different tubes. Because the radioactivity is distributed in the patient a large piece of lead with many small holes (collimator) is used so that only radiation traveling to the detector along specific lines is detected (Fig. 8.2).

Nuclear medicine also has its CT scanner. Those that use the more common radionuclides, such as technetium-99m, which emit only one γ-rays (or photon) at a time, are referred to as SPECT. Some radionuclides, such as fluorine-18, emit positrons, which annihilate themselves when they come in contact with an electron. These positron emitters produce two photons that travel in opposite directions. These are detected by a ring of detectors similar to those in X-ray CT in a process called positron emission tomography (PET). Positron emitters have very short lives and have to be used shortly after they are produced. Thus, PET scanners have to be relatively close to a high-energy linear accelerator used to produce the radionuclides (Fig. 8.3).

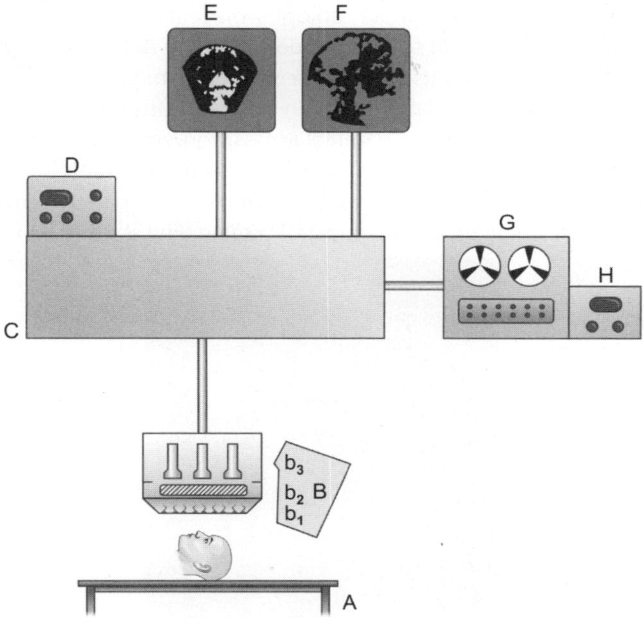

Fig. 8.2: The nuclear medicine image (NMI) profile specifies basic display capabilities that are required in nuclear medicine

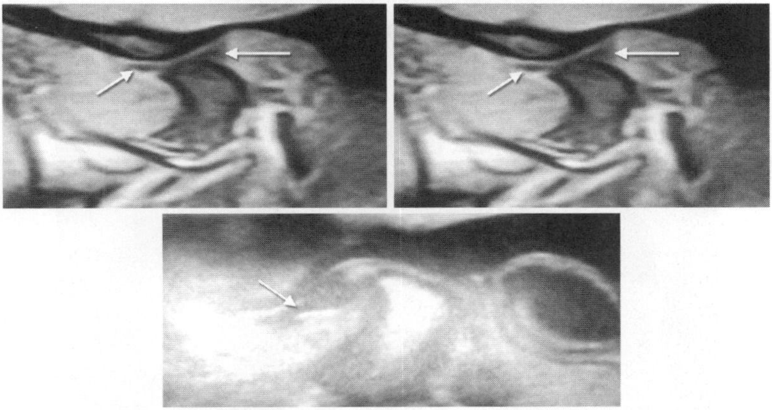

Fig. 8.3: Images of temporomandibular joint—showing articular disk

By selecting the appropriate radiopharmaceutical, one can target a specific part or location of the body. Soon after the radiopharmaceutical is administered, it makes its way to the target organ, bone or tissue. The radioisotope serves as a label that can be traced inside the body. The patient is examined under a gamma or positron emission tomography camera, which displays an image of the organ on the screen. The doctor interprets these images to determine the source of the patient's problem. This procedure is known as a diagnostic imaging (Figs 8.4 and 8.5).

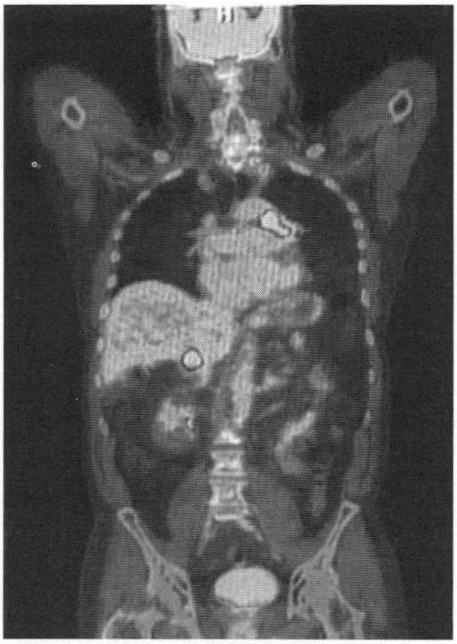

Fig. 8.4: Preparing the patient for cardiac nuclear medicine

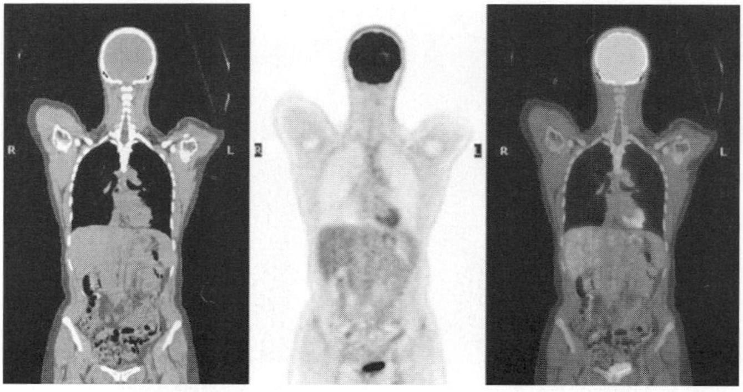

Fig. 8.5: PET scanning—used in nuclear medicine to obtain pictures of the metabolic (functional) activity within particular areas of the body

BONE SCANNING

Bone scanning is one of the most frequently performed nuclear medicine studies. Bone scans can be used to diagnose and differentiate osteomyelitis from cellulitis, as well as detect primary and metastatic malignant disease. They can also be used to assess the vascularity of bone grafts and contribute to the diagnosis of various metabolic bone diseases such as fibrous displasia, Paget's disease, osteoarthritis, and rheumatoid arthritis. Basic advantage of bone scan is that one can detect 10–15% mineral loss, while standard radiographs will only visualize a bony defect after 30–50% mineral loss. Overall scan has a high sensitivity but low specificity.

The bone scan uses a technetium-99 m methylene diphosphonate with a half-life of 6 hours and a total radiation dose of 0.3 rads. It is thought the diphosphonate molecule is taken up by in areas of increased osteoblastic activity and vascularity (Fig. 8.6).

The metabolic activity of the osteoblasts incorporates calcium phosphate during the process of ossification. It is thought the diphosphonate molecule accumulates in the area of increased osteoblastic activity as it binds to calcium ions to form calcium phosphate. The normal bone scan should demonstrate symmetry around the midline with uniform uptake of the radiopharmaceutical (Fig. 8.7). There is usually increased activity at joint margins and vertebral bodies. Uptake is typically visualized in the kidneys and bladder.

To obtain additional diagnostic information, a three-phase bone scan is performed especially to distinguish osteomyelitis from cellulitis.

1. The dynamic vascular flow phase, where imaging is performed every 2 to 3 seconds for the first 30 seconds. In this phase, each side can be compared and differences in vascularity can be seen.

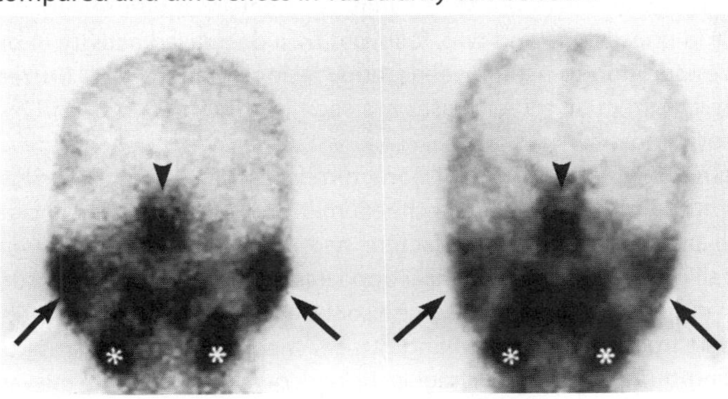

Fig. 8.6: Uptake of radionuclide material

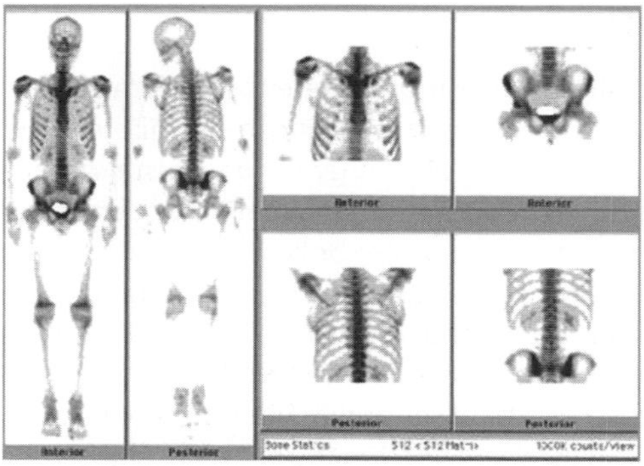

Fig. 8.7: Normal bone scanning image

2. The blood pool image at 5 minutes, where the radiopharmaceutical is mostly in the vascular compartment but is starting to appear bone. This phase demonstrates regional differences in blood flow and vascular permeability.
3. Two to four hours later, the osseous delayed static image is obtain usually for the entire body demonstrating regional distribution in the skeleton. This phase reflects the metabolic activity of the bone in question. In non-inflammatory condition, the third phase is the only image obtained.

Occasionally, a fourth-phase study is performed 24 hours later when there may be improved contrast between normal bone and inflammatory condition. In osteomyelitis there is abnormal accumulation of the radiopharmaceutical in all three phases, with a more focal bony uptake in the third and fourth phases. Cellulitis presents as a diffusely increased uptake in phases one and two, followed by a decreased activity in phase three. In addition to osteomyelitis, bony lesions that are "hot" (increased accumulation) in all three phases are seen in acute fractures and hyper-vascular tumors.

Both benign and malignant bone tumors as well as metastatic lesions demonstrate increase uptake of technetium-99 m. However, areas of increased uptake are nonspecific, since a facture, neoplastic lesion and inflammatory lesion all produce images of similar appearance. Metabolic diseases such as fibrous dysplasia and Paget's disease also show increased uptake on the scan.

Apart from the bone scanning nuclear medicine imaging is useful for detecting, tumors, aneurysm, irregular or inadequate blood flow to the various tissues, and blood cell disorders and inadequate functioning of the organs.

SALIVARY GLAND SCANNING

Pertechnetate (99m Tc04-) is concentrated and excreted by several glandular tissues, including mammary, thyroid, and salivary glands. It is an excellent procedure to study salivary gland functions and pathophysiology. As salivary gland scans can be evaluated visually or may be quantitated with the help of a computer, a strong baseline of normal studies can be generated, and subsequent scans may provide useful information in the diagnosis of a variety of pathophysiologic condition.

A salivary gland scan usually consists of a dynamic or flow study followed by a static study, and takes 30–60 minutes to perform. While the patient's nose is against the imaging head, 5 to 10 mCi of 99m Tc04- are injected intravenously. This is called the anterior position and results in an anterior view. Multiple images are taken during the first 30–120 seconds, that show the flow of blood first into the arterial and venous systems of the head and neck and then into the organs of the region. This constitutes the flow study portion of the examination. It yields information on the vascularity of the area and on any functional vascular abnormalities that may be associated with the salivary gland. During the next 30–40 minutes, sequential "static" image are taken by moving/shifting the patient head in left and right lateral, anterior, and sometime posterior position, which demonstrate the anatomy of the major salivary glands and their ability to produce and secrete saliva. Finally, the patient is to given a sialagogue, such as lemon juice or citric acid, to stimulate the flow of saliva. A final series of static images is then taken to demonstrate the stimulated secretory capabilities of the gland.

Reports of salivary scanning on patients with salivary gland infections are scarce because the diagnosis is usually made on the basis of history and clinical observation. Never the less, scans may be useful in acute inflammation because sialography is usually contraindicated in such cases. Acute inflammation generally results in increased tracer uptake and a visually "hot" or dense salivary gland image. This is thought to be caused by hyperemia and vascular stasis in the gland. Chronic recurrent infections often lead to progressive fibrotic obliteration of functional parenchyma, which results in glandular atrophy and decreased tracer uptake by the gland giving a visually non-dense or "cold" salivary gland image.

Sjögren's syndrome, an autoimmune disease in which salivary gland function is partially or completely destroyed, is particularly suitable for evaluation by salivary gland scanning. Because of the progressive nature of the loss of salivary function in such patients, salivary gland scans have proved extremely useful, not only in determining the severity of the disease but also in following the response of salivary gland function to antinflammatory chemotherapy.

Salivary gland neoplasm's are most troublesome entities to diagnose because of the difficulty of salivary gland, biopsy the dangers of injury to the seventh cranial nerve, the high incidence of malignancy in submandibular gland tumors, and the short comings of conventional radiologic examinations. The unique biologic characteristics of various salivary gland tumors led to the hope that 99m Tc04- might demonstrate specificity for tumors in which it would not concentrate. Although warthin's tumor almost invariably concentrates 99m Tc04- and metastasis lesions are almost invariably devoid of the tracer the overall results of tumor scans have unfortunately been inconsistent.

POSITRON EMMISSION TOMOGRAPHY

Positron emmission tomography (PET) also known as positron computed tomography (PCT) or physiologic tomography is a cross-sectional imaging technique delineates internal structures and permits the measurement of local biochemical processes.

Positron imaging is accomplished by administering a physiologically active compound labeled with a positron-emitting isotope (11C. 18F. 13N. 15O). The post injection distribution of the isotopes determined by an appropriate detection system and a two-dimensional image is mathematically constructed. The image reflects the distribution of the traged compound. For example, if an area of a tissue or organ that normally activity metabolized a compound is found to be free of tracer it is apparent that abnormality exists. This can be determined noninvasive by PET.

In PET when a position is obtained from the radioactive decay, it rapidly encounters a free electron combines with it and both disappear; they are said to be annihilated. When they combine their masses, they are converted into electromagnetic energy in the form of two annihilation photons, each with 511 key energy. The decay is unique in that the two photons are emitted in opposite direction from the point of annihilation; their paths are said to be coincident.

This permits a pair of coincident scintillator in a ring of detector around the patient to determine the trajectory of the photons. This is called annihilation coincidence detection. If only one detector in a pair detects a photon, it is apparent that the event took place outside the well-defined region surveyed by that pair so it is electronically rejected. After data are accumulated from a large number of events along the lines through pairs of coincident detectors and at many discrete angles through 180° a matrix of unknown representing a cross-sectional plane through the object can be solved and a tomographic image can be mathematically constructed. The mathematical model is the same as that used in X-ray CT.

Clinically useful applications of PET have been in the investigation of liver, pituitary gland, brain, heart, thyroid, adrenal gland.

The radiation exposures of the patient resulting from PET are much lower than for conventional nuclear medicine technique. Unfortunately, the useful isotope have short or very short half lives so that the PRT equipment can only be sited close to a cyclotron which limits considerably the availably of this useful technique.

RADIOCHEMICAL STABILITY AND STORAGE

Stability (shelf-life) of radiolabeled compound is determined by a combination of the chemical and radiochemical decomposition processes. Radiochemical compounds with high specific activities are more likely to undergo radiation-include chemical degradation. Tritium products are generally less stable then the carbon 14 products. This is due to the fact that tritium compounds usually have a much higher specific activity and are generally stored at low chemical concentrations (mg/mL) in solution. This is particularly a problem for aqueous and saline solutions, where non-sterile conditions can lead to microbial degradation.

Proper storage of radiochemical compound is important. Product information sheet is provided with each product, which give the recommended storage condition. Product are rigorously tested, and then re-analyzed approximately every 6-month to ensure that the purity specification are met. This provides with the highest quality product available. General methods for analysis include HPLC, GC, and gel electrophoresis with electronic radioimaging, with HPLC being the preferred method for analysis.

9 Temporomandibular Joint Imaging

The diagnosis and treatment of temporomandibular disorders remains one of the most challenging areas of dentistry. With the newly expanded diagnostic imaging capability, the clinician must determine which technique offers the highest probability of significantly aiding diagnosis and treatment.

Advances in both the diagnostic and the understanding of the underlying mechanism of dysfunction of temperomandibular joint (TMJ) have been made possible by recent developments in imaging. Imaging procedures may be subdivided into the examination of the osseous components and the soft tissue components of the joint. Examination of the bone usually precedes that of the soft tissue. Omission of the osseous component may eliminate significant information.

The osseous investigations provide information of the shape and internal structure of the condylar head and neck and temporal bone; and to illustrate the relationship of the condyle to the glenoid fossa and articular eminence in mandibular open and close positions. The following modalities can fulfill these needs: pantomography, transpharyngeal view, transorbital view (or open townie's), and open and close transcranial views.

These conventional techniques still provide information that may not be apparent in advanced imaging modalities. Because of relatively low cost and low patient exposure to radiation, these techniques provide an adequate initial level of investigation. When required, more sophisticated imaging methods such as tomography, computed tomography (CT), cone beam computed tomography (CBCT) and nuclear imaging may be applied.

The second stage of investigation may include the assessment of the soft tissue component of the joint. Advanced imaging techniques permit the direct examination of the articular disk. Disorders such as abnormalities in position, shape, and internal structure of the disk may be detected through the use of arthrography and magnetic resonance imaging (MRI).

TOMOGRAPHY

The two types of tomographic machines commonly used for the joint are linear and poly directional machines (e.g. hypocycloidal). Both are capable of producing images of diagnostic quality. The polydirectional machines, however can achieve a better blurring effect of structures of on either side of tomographic slice. It is not known whether the streaking evidence in images from linear machines obscures a significant amount of information. The quality of lateral joint images may be improved significantly by correcting the horizontal angle of the central ray so that the tomographic slices are at right angles to the long axis of the condylar head. Most technique involves measuring of the angle of the condylar head to the midsagittal plane in the basal skull view. If this view is not available, 15° to 20° rotation of the head toward the examined side will improve the image. The same technique may be applied to anteroposterior views. Lateral tomographic slices should provide a series of images that include the most extreme medial and lateral aspects of the joint. The size of image should be enlarged when considering abnormalities of the coronoid process.

Indications

Tomography is used to access condylar positions and to supplement further detail of the bone structure. Tomograph can provide true lateral views of the joint by blurring the image of overlapping osseous structures that obscure the joint in convectional radiography. In this fashion, a more accurate representation of the condylar position within the fossa (joint space) can be obtained, because the shape of the condyle does not duplicate the often irregular shape of the fossa, the condyle may appear to have different positions in the medial and lateral aspects of the joint. This suggest that a three-dimensional analysis of the joint space may be required. Actual measurements of the joint space may be of limited value as there is a significant variation in the normal population also; posterior positioning of the condyle does not appear to have a statistically significant predictive value for the diagnosis of disk displacement. By eliminating overlapping structure, tomography may reveal osseous changes that are not apparent in conventional films, especially in the medial aspect of the joint. This imaging method may reveal small erosions or small osteophytes characteristic of degenerative joint disease. Also it is valuable in defining the extent of bone involvement with arthritis or the presence of neoplasm.

Limitations

Tomographic blurring will decrease the sharpness of image and this may obscure small changes. A bone surface that curves sharply, such as the most medial and lateral aspect of the condyle will not be reproduced with sufficient detail. These deficiencies however, may be eliminated when tomograph are used in combinations with conventional radiography.

COMPUTED TOMOGRAPHY

Sagittal slices of the joint may be obtained by reformatting the information from the axial slice or by attempting to obtain direct sagittal slices. The direct acquisition of sagittal slices may be limited by the equipment and patient flexibility but will provide superior images. If is not possible to acquire sagittal images, then the minimum requirement would be both axial and coronal images. A three-dimensional image can be constructed by a mathematical manipulation of the data derived from a series of slices.

Cone Beam Computed Tomography

Role of cone beam computed tomography (CBCT), for dental and maxillofacial diagnostic osseous tasks has been rapidly developed as an alternative to conventional CT for assessment of the TMJ, CBCT results in images of CT-like quality, yet is made with less expensive equipment and components, shorter patient examination time, and much lower radiation dose than required for conventional CT.

The introduction of the CBCT technology specifically designed for use in dentistry has opened up new opportunities in TMJ imaging. CBCT has been recognized as a reliable method for the examination of the osseous components of the TMJ.

CBCT provides images that can be reconstructed in planes parallel or perpendicular to the long axis of the condyle instead of the true anatomic coronal and sagittal planes. This results in high quality images of the bony components in all planes. Because the patients are positioned in a relatively natural head position, the TMJ positional relationships can be more accurately evaluated than in a CT examination where the patient is supine.

Indication

CT would be used when a greater amount of detail about the form and internal structure of the osseous component is requier. Attempts at imaging the articular disk using soft-tissue window imaging have not been successful when compared with arthrography or MR imaging.

The strength of these digital images lies in the capability of revealing small bone detail such as erosions or small sequestra within the condylar head. The extent of tumor involvement of the surrounding soft tissues or osseous structures. Other uses includes demonstration of contact between a hyperplasic coronoid process and the inside of the zygomatic arch. Also, the extent of any alkalosis can be revealed. Three-dimensional reformatted images can help with preoperative perception of the extent of disease and, in the future, possible with the reconstruction of joints.

Limitations

Although in specific instances CT may reveal more bone detail then tomography, in general, both imaging modalities appear to be comparable. Also, conventional tomography is less costly and delivers a smaller absorbed dose of radiation.

SCINTIGRAPHY

Radioactive elements such as technetium-99m are injected intravenously and the accumulation of this radiopharmaceutical agent within various tissues of the body is monitored with a gamma cemera. Technetium-99m will accumulate where bone is being formed and where there is increased vascularity. Gallium will accumulate where there is an active infection.

Indications

Technetium-99m is used to detect an abnormal increase in bone formation within the joint such as a bone-forming tumor, infection, or degenerative joint disease. This imaging modality also has been employed to monitor the presence or absence of active growth in case of condylar hyperplasia. Abnormal activity within the condyle may indicate degenerative or remodeling activity instead of active growth.

A diagnosis of septic arthritis may be confirmed when both technetium-99m and gallium scans reveal abnormal accumulation.

Limitations

The results of technetium scans are nonspecific because many conditions can stimulate bone formation. The inability to provide absolute quantification limits their use.

ARTHROGRAPHY

This procedure involves the injection of a radiopaque contrast fluid into the joint spaces to provide an indirect image of the articular disk. To obtain an acceptable image of the disk, both the inferior and superior joint spaces must be injected. This procedure should be done under fluoroscopic observation to reduce morbidity and maximize the diagnostic benefit. By observing the flow of contrast, perforations, discontinuities in the joint capsule, and adhesions can be observed. Once both spaces are injected, a dynamic study of the movement of the disk during jaw movements can be made and recorded. Subsequently to the injections, tomography can provide further detail of the morphology of the disk.

Double—contrast image entail the removal of the contrast fluid from the spaces and the injection of air. This provides an increased contrast in the tomographic images as the radiolucent air sharply contrast with the surrounding soft tissues that are saturated with contrast medium.

Indications

Arthrography provides information regarding the soft-tissue components, specifically the shape and position of the articular disk. Fluoroscopic observation of the injection may reveal the presence of adhesion, perforation, and discontinuities in the capsule and provide dynamic study of disk movement. Also, any abnormal accumulation of joint fluid will be evident. It has been demonstrated that with the addition of tomography, the diagnosis of abnormalities in the position and the shape of the disk is accurate. The most frequent displacement is anterior or anteromedial. Anteromedial rotation may be diagnosed by carefully evaluating the lateral to medial tomographic image. Direct medial or lateral displacement is difficult to interpret with this image modility. The high frequency of anterior displacement has challenged the present concept of normal variation.

The accepted normal disk position in the mandibular closed position presents the posterior band in a superior position to the condylar head and the intermediate zone of the disk position to act as the articulating surface between the anterosuperior condylar surface and the articular eminence. Number of patient with anterior disk positioned are asymptomatic. Deformed disk have been described as biconvex, bilinear, or with an enlarge posterior band. Also, normal variation such as large anterior band may result in the misdiagnosis of disk displacement.

Limitations

This imaging procedure is not proficient in identifying direct medial or lateral disk displacements and sometime present difficulty when disk is severely deformed. Unlike MRI, this procedure has an associated morbidity and exposure to ionizing radiation. It also declines in use in light of increased availability of MR imaging.

MAGNETIC RESONANCE IMAGING

Superior anatomic details are provided by using T1-weighted images. Other techniques of choice use proton-weighted images and sometime includes T2-weighted images for the detection of abnormal fluid accumulation. There is benefit to directing the sagittal slice at right angles to the long axis of the condylar head and including coronal image. A reduction in slice thickness from 3–1.5 mm has been proposed to increase image quality.

Indications

Similar to arthrography, MRI is ordered to provide information about the shape and position of the articular disk. The articular disk is identified by its biconcave morphology and by the fact that the signal from the disk differs from the surrounding tissue. The accuracy in determining the disk position and morphology is comparable to arthrography. It is difficult to identify the disk when it is grossly deformed.

In normal circumstances, the margin between the low signal of the posterior band and the high signal of the bilaminar ligament is identified easily. After the disk is displaced, the bilaminar ligament now serving as the articulating surface may fibrotic, resulting in a lower signal that may become indistinguishable from the disk.

MRI can detected abnormal changes within the disk. Myxomatous degeneration of the disk resulting in a higher tissue signal. Whereas abnormally low signal from the cancellous portion of the condylar head, which has been interpreted as avascular necrosis. It may be difficult, however, to differentiate this from sclerosis that results from degenerative joint disease. Abnormal joint fluid may be detected by T2-weighted images.

Limitations

Changes in the tissue signal may hamper disk identification. MRI modality cannot diagnose perforation or adhesions and does not provide a dynamic study. Substantial cost and availability may pose problems.

10 Digital Subtraction Radiography

Transmission radiographs contain more information than can readily be seen by eye. Background structures such as the alveolar bone and adjacent teeth may draw the examiner's vision away from the diagnostic information, thereby making detection of pathologic changes difficult. In the diagnosis of periodontal disease, an existing level of alveolar bone loss is readily visible, but the progression of the bone loss from one radiographic examination to the next may be very difficult to interpret.

Further, the visualization of furcation involvement may be obscured by overlap of tooth roots. The advancement of caries from an incipient lesion through the dentoenamel junction is often difficult to detect. The detection of initial saucering or formation of an angular defect around implants is very difficult to visualize on radiographs. Moreover, the spread of bone loss along threads of a root form implant is often obscured by the sharp contrast between the bone and the implant surface.

Subtraction radiography addresses many of the limitations in the detection of these radiographic changes by decreasing the amount of distracting background information and by allowing the eye to focus on the actual change that has occurred between two images. By subtracting all the anatomic structures that have not changed between radiographic examinations, changes in diagnostic information are easier. Technically, this as an image enhancement method the removes the structured noise from the images. The result is the area of change clearly displayed either against a neutral gray background or superimposed on the original radiograph itself. The subtraction of the two original radiographs is termed an image rather than a radiograph, because it does not directly result from exposure of a radiographic film.

There are two major limitations to subtraction imaging with photographic methods. These are the inability to correct projection geometry and density and contrast of the radiographic film.

It is important to remember that digitization does not increase the information available over that contained in the original radiograph. Actually, digitization decreases the information content but turns the image into a form that can be read and analyzed by the computer. It is this computer analysis that gives digital subtraction radiography (DSR) its ability to accurately display differences between images that are too small to be seen by the unaided human eye.

To obtain a subtraction image using a hypothetical perfect set of radiographs, specialized computer software is used. The first radiograph is digitized and turned into a positive image in the computer. The software then allows the operator to align the second radiograph under the video camera. When alignment is complete, the second radiograph is digitized. The computer then subtracts the digitized gray-scale value at each grid or pixel location to obtain the subtraction image. At this point, a perfect subtraction with no difference between images will have a value of zero (black) in all pixel locations. To facilitate visualization, an offset gray value of 128 is added to produce a gray background against which any superimposed change or lesion is more readily visible. The interpretation of this ideal subtraction may be muted by the fact that the teeth and other anatomic features have been subtracted and are therefore, not visible. This could be a problem in determining the exact location of a lesion.

To circumvent this problem, the software can superimpose a color-coded lesion on the original radiograph. Three methods have been employed in the recent literature to achieve this result. The first is the use of a bite registration and film holder attached to the radiographic source. The second method uses extraoral stabilization of the patient and long source-to-object distance to minimize magnification effects. The patient's head is stabilized with a cephalostat during exposure. The third method uses a stored video image of the patient's face taken during the first radiographic examination to align the patient for subsequent exposures. This last method is versatile and is applicable to extraoral imaging but requires significantly more equipment than the prior techniques.

The particular importance in oral imaging is the change in density or contrast that may occur in serial radiographic images. Density and contrast changes caused by fluctuations in the line voltage, exposure settings of film, or processing may lead to variations in the overall density and contrast of the image. As the assessment of alveolar bone gain or loss is made by subtracting the gray levels of two images to isolate changes that have occurred, subtraction methods require that the film pairs have nearly identical density and contrast. The matching of the density and contrast of the two films commonly is done by employing a contrast correction algorithm.The computer programs match the gray level distribution of subsequent images to the gray levels found in the original reference image. In this way, small changes in density and contrast over time may be corrected retrospectively using digital image processing.

DSR may be used not only for the assessment of the progression of periodontal disease but also for healing in response to therapy. DSR has been applied to the evaluation of implant success and failure and the assessment of caries progression and remineralization. Moreover, DSR may have a role in the diagnosis and evaluation of temporomandibular. DSR continues to show promise for the diagnosis and evaluation of the results of therapy for a wide range of dental diseases (Figs 10.1A to C).

IMAGE SUBTRACTION

Since there is so much information on a conventional radiography diagnostically important may be difficult to identify if they are small. This is an important consideration since the detection and/or successful treatment of number of dental diseases depends upon the early recognition of small changes in tissue density. For example, periodontist need in the radiograph minute lesions in the interproximal bone, buccal and lingual bony plates and tabular bone at the bifurcation and trifurcation. Obviously the task of

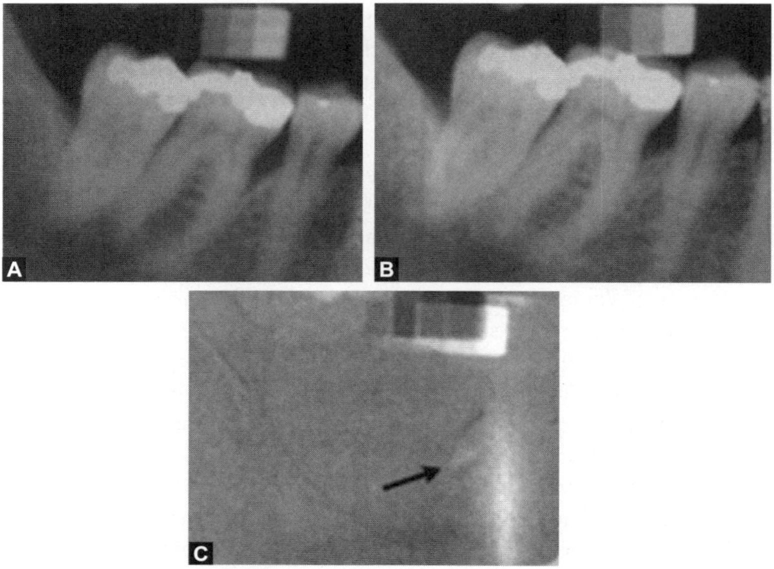

Figs 10.1A to C: (A) Baseline image; (B) Standardized 1-year follow-up image; (C) Subtraction image showing increase in bone

diagnostician would be easier and efficient if all the unwanted information could be eliminated from the film. The image subtraction dose just that; it is photographic method that eliminates unwanted image from a radiograph and makes diagnostic important information easier to see.

Image subtraction is accomplished by subtracting one photograph from another. First a SCOUT' film is made and after changes takes place in the tissue under study, a second radiograph is made. If the image on the first radiograph could be subtracted from the second all that would remain would be the changes. This is accomplished by making a negative film of the " SCOUT".

Film on which everything that was white is now black and blacks white. However at the negative copy of the SCOUT film is superimposed with the second film, everything on the two films will be invisible except tissue changes that has occurred and that is quite apparent. Although changes are not at a high contrast, they are quite apparent and quite good information relative to the position of the change, the superimposed image can be reviewed over a film illuminator or subtraction photograph can be made.

This technique has some difficulties; it is necessary to have the patient completely motionless when the radiographs are made. In both the radiograph patients position and radiation source should be same, it is also necessary to exactly superimpose the second film with the negative of the SCOUT film.

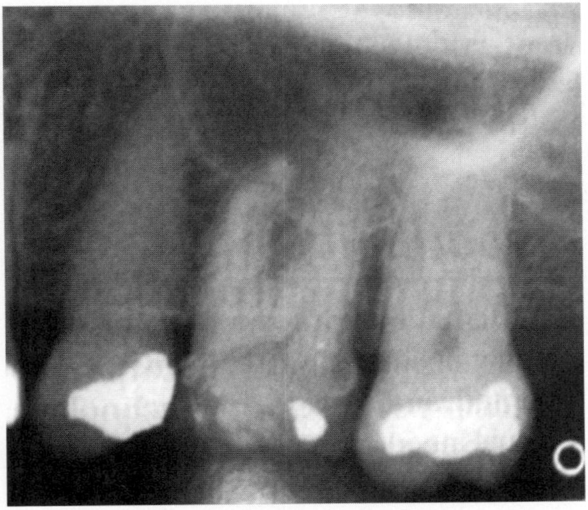

Fig. 10.2: Measurement tool to determine the length of crown and root of the molar

Electronic subtraction is also currently possible by taking advantage of the television systems capabilities of addition, subtraction and storing image.

APPLICATIONS

1. Study of the periodontal diseases and progression of therapy.
2. Sialography.
3. To evaluate results of root canal therapy (Fig. 10.2).

11 Radiovisiography

The X-ray is being used as most important diagnostic aid since their discovery in 1895 to record various structures of diagnostic importance on the silver halide coated polyester films. At present virtually there is no challenge as an image receptor to these films for the intraoral radiograph.

Though the sensitivity of these films has been increased to a very high degree, they have two major disadvantages. A fairly high radiation dose and wet film processing interrupting the treatment. To overcome these disadvantages a new rapid digital imaging system, radiovisiography (RVG) has been introduced in dentistry. RVG was invented in 1989 by MOUYEN in France. It presents intraoral radiographic image immediately after the exposure.

Radiovisiography (RVG) is depending on the CCD (charge coupled device) technique, i.e. electronic imaging by video camera. The CCD is a solid-state detector array with metal oxide such as silicon semiconductor structure that is extremely sensitive to electromagnetic radiation. These CCD detectors are used in video cameras, microscope, astronomers telescope, radiographic imaging.

COMPONENTS OF RADIOVISIOGRAPHY

The RVG system comprises of four main components:

- Dental X-ray machine with a specific timer
- Intraoral sensor
- Display processing unit
- Printer.

Dental X-ray Machine with a Specific Timer

The X-ray generator is of conventional type but it is provided with special electronic timer (ccx) to give accurately controlled short exposure times required.

Intraoral Sensor

The primary image receptor in the sensor is a rare-earth intensifying screen (25 mm × 16 mm) housed in a rigid plastic casing (40.6 mm long × 22.8 mm wide × 14 mm thick), behind which is an array of optical fibers.

During an exposure, when the X-rays are incident upon it, intensifying screen fluoresces and that light is conducted by optical fiber to a CCD. The CCD detects the pattern of light and translates into electrical signals which are received by display processing units through a long flexible cable connecting the sensor to the display processing unit.

The intraoral sensor is anatomically adopted to fit in proper position inside the oral cavity. Its edges and angel's are rounded to avoid the injury to the oral soft tissue.

As the sensor can not be sterilized, it is covered during use by a disposable latex finger sheath. The sensor can be held in the mouth by the patient, by a bite block attachment or by using one of a range of specially designed sensor-holding, bean aiming devices (Fig. 11.1).

Display Processing Units

The display unit digitizes, processes and stores the analog signals coming from the CCD. It has also got the television screen on which the images are displayed. When an exposure is made instantly an image appears on the left hand side of the TV screen with a four-fold magnification of the primary image. If needed, image from second exposure may then by displayed on the right hand side of the screen without loss of the first image. The display

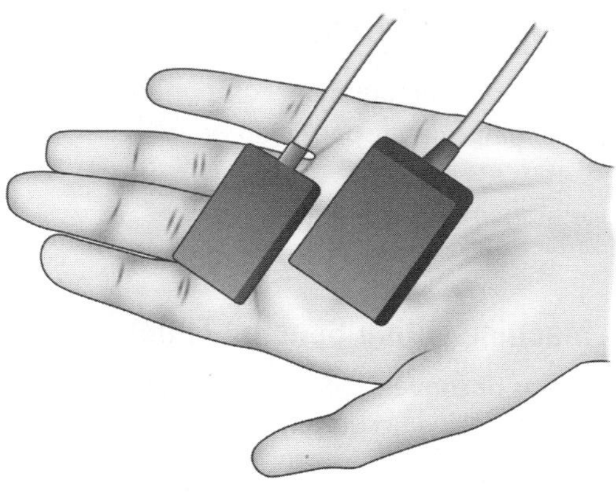

Fig. 11.1: Intraoral sensor

processing unit allows manipulation of image like enhancement of the image, contrast stretching and positive to negative conversion. The original image can be stored in the unit and can be called on the screen at any time.

It is also provided with a zoom feature to produce an enlargement of any part of image present on the screen for a detailed study, this is particularly helpful to study the initial periapical changes (Fig. 11.2).

Printer

A separate dry silver printer is used to produce permanent record of the images present on the TV screen. This produces hard copy images similar in appearance to black and white photographic prints, which are slightly smaller than the TV screen images.

APPLICATIONS OF RVG

The RVG system is capable of producing images of diagnostic value. It shows whole tooth along with its surrounding bone, hence application of RVG are similar to intraoral periapical-ray used, mainly for periodontal pathosis.

Radiovisiography is a rapid imaging system that can produce clinically acceptable periapical image at a lower radiation dose then conventional intraoral radiography. Image quality appears to be adequate for clinical use and image distortion is minimal. It is believed that RVG represent a significant development in the field of dental radiography.

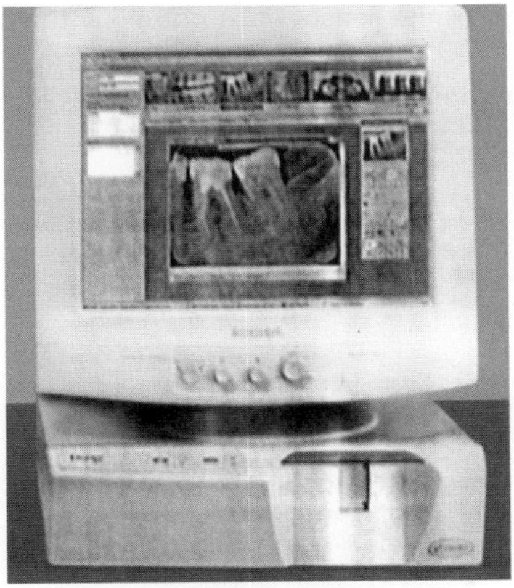

Fig. 11.2: Digora FMX system

Advantages of RVG

- It is a rapid imaging system, which produces the image almost immediately after the exposure.
- The required dose is low due to reduction in exposure by 70–80%.
- As this system does not requires X-ray films it does not involve any processing.
- The image resolution is adequate for all the clinical applications.
- It produces images with minimal inherent distortion compared to conventional film radiography.
- It provides facilities for image manipulation like enhancement, brightness and contrast control and positive to negative conversion.
- It can be linked to a computer for storage of the images, which can be called on the screen at any time helping the clinician to compare the two radiographs taken at intervals.
- It also helps in patient's education by showing him pre- and post-operative status.

Disadvantages of RVG

- The X-ray sensitive surface of the sensor can accommodate only one molar or two incisors at time. Hence if peripical images of several adjacent teeth are required, a greater number of RVG images are needed compared to conventional intraoral radiographs.
- Size and form of the sensor does not allow the occlusal bitewing projections.
- The bulk of intraoral sensor sometimes causes difficult for placement of sensor.

12 Implant Radiology

The key to success of any surgical implant procedure is the preoperative planning. Case selection involves clinical assessment of the site(s) by visual examination and appropriate radiographic imaging. Other factors such as selection of the appropriate implant, patient education, patient preparation and risk estimation for procedure are also necessary components to successful implant. The role of radiography in the presurgical, intratreatment and post placement phases are outlined, as well as the advantages and limitations of each imaging modality.

PRESURGICAL RADIOGRAPHIC EVALUATION

Periapical, Occlusal and Panoramic Techniques

Radiographic evaluation in this phase of implant techniques should help the clinician determine:

1. The quantity of bone present.
2. The quality of bone available.
3. The location of critical anatomic structures. Generally, it is sound practice to obtain multiple views of the proposed site to assess adequately the height and width of the bone. This may mandate the use of several imaging techniques.

For a single site therefore it would be necessary to take several periapical radiographs and at least one properly positioned and exposed occlusal radiograph. These films probably afford the best image detail of the site with minimal geometric distortion. Intraoral radiographs are useful to help determine the approximate height of the bone as well as the distance of the proposed site from anatomic structures such as the mental and incisive foramina, maxillary sinus, inferior alveolar nerve, and the incisive and canine fossae. The use of an occlusal film taken at 90° to the mandibular dental arch would give excellent information about the buccolingual width of the bone. The shape or architecture of the bone in three-dimensions, however, is not always apparent on an occlusal film, especially in the posterior mandible. An occlusal view of the maxillary arch is often distorted and may be less useful for arch width determination. Therefore, additional views such as tomographs, may be required for adequate assessment.

These intraoral films, together with panaromic radiograph, can reveal information about bone quality such as density, trabecular pattern and presence of anomalies in the proposed region. Additionally, panoramic radiograph, if properly positioned, are useful adjuncts for even single implant site selection because they allow comparison to contralateral structures. They also may reveal problems such as odontogenic lesions, condylar changes and so on at remote sites that could jeopardize the implant placement or prognosis. Panoramic films are also useful for a preliminary look at multiple implant sites.

Nevertheless, panoramic radiology as the sole means of radiographic presurgical assessment is inappropriate because the technique is extremely sensitive to errors in patient position. Several authors have outlined these errors and their corrections.

A great majority of articles in the literature that deals with implants show pre- or postoperative panoramic images that have distortion due to one or more positioning errors. If clinician continues to use only this imaging technique for implant assessment, they must be trained sufficiently in panoramic radiology to understand its limitations. If not, the risk potential litigation problems because of inadequate radiographic assessment that may contribute to failure of the prosthesis.

In addition to the myriad of possible positioning errors, the use of panoramic films alone may lead to errors in estimating or determining the bone width. Although most clinicians who place implants can assess the bone width clinically at the time of surgery, several other imaging modalities—plain tomography, CT, and three-dimensional CT reconstructions—are available to help the clinician visualize the anatomy of the proposed site to avoid potential problems.

INTRAORAL IMAGING USING ELECTRONIC OR CCD IMAGING

Technique

With the introduction of charge-coupled devices (CCDs), presurgical implant assessment of single sites may become more precise. Area array, solid-state detectors (CCDs) may allow more accurate measurement of implant sites preoperatively and provide more information about osseointegration postoperatively than has been available with film. The use of wire grids with known geometric size will help clinicians with site selection and height determination (Figs 12.1 and 12.2).

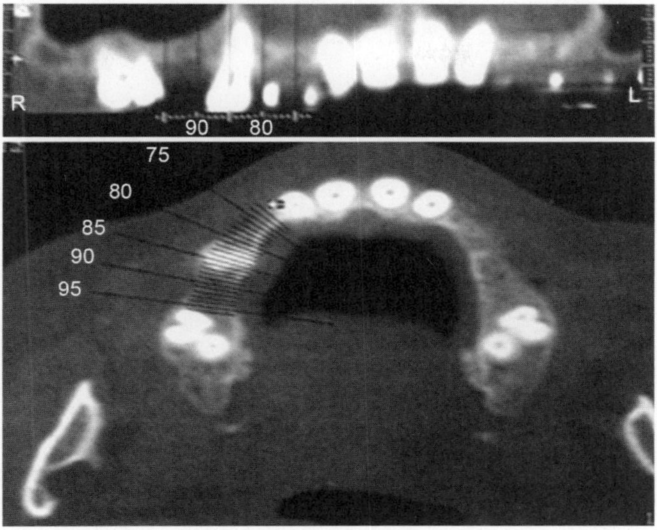

Fig. 12.1A: Reformatted CT study of the maxilla using 3-D Dental software. Axial and panoramic-like curved linear reconstructed image using an imaging stent incorporating gutta-percha marker

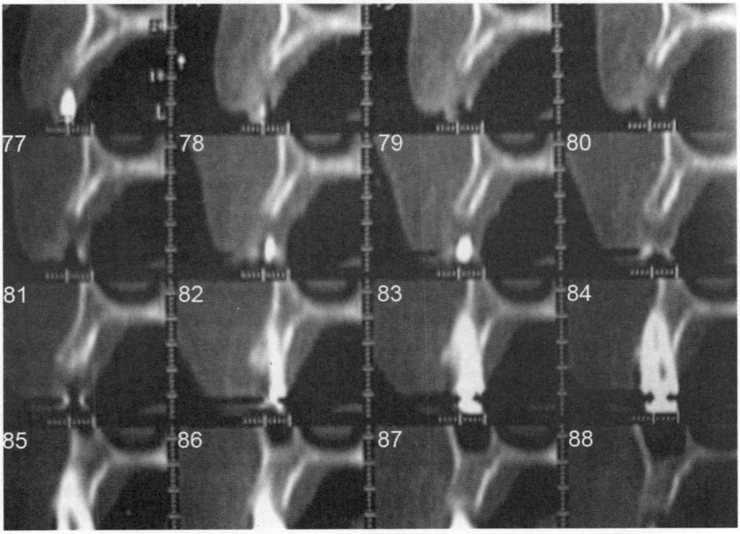

Fig. 12.1B: Reformatted CT study of the maxilla using 3-D Dental software. Cross-sectional images that correlate with the image in A

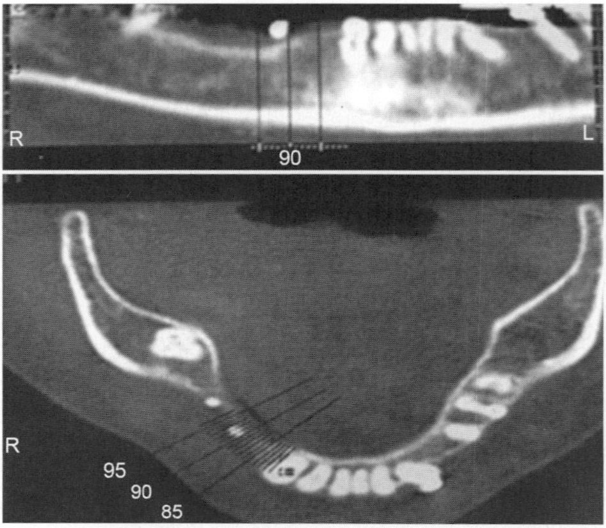

Fig. 12.2A: Reformatted CT study of the mandible using 3-D Dental software. Axial and panoramic-like curved linear reconstructed image using an imaging stent incorporating gutta-percha marker

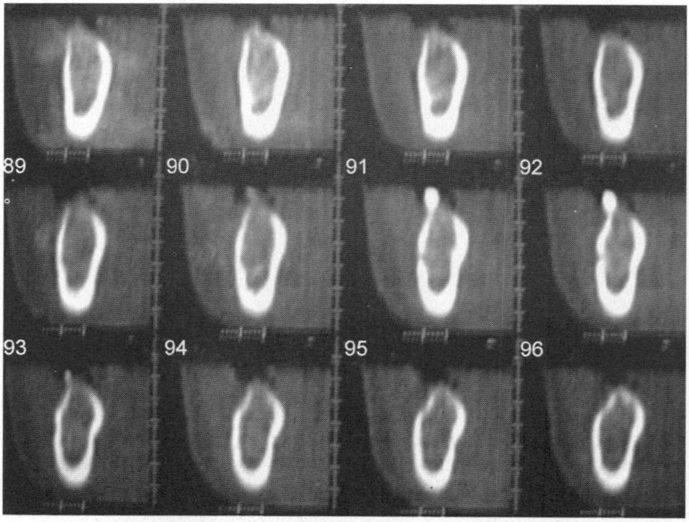

Fig. 12.2B: Reformatted CT study of the mandible using 3-D Dental software. Cross-sectional images that correlate with the image in A

As computers are integrated into imaging process, software will be developed to compare accurately and automatically a grid and implant to the anatomic site. Multiple images of a proposed site may lead eventually to two- and three-dimensional reconstruction of the proposed implant site and allow the dentist to view the information on a video monitor prior to placement, not unlike some of the CT images currently available at greater expense.

TOMOGRAPHIC TECHNIQUES

The most cost-effective method of radiographic assessment of implant sites is probably plain film tomography, either linear or multidirectional. Plain tomography refers to the simultaneous movement of the X-ray tube and X-ray film in opposite directions to produce a slice or selected image layer in which there is increased contrast and resolution of the structures of interest. In the linear tomography, the film and X-ray tube pass in opposite directions, in a horizontal and vertical manner, through an imaginary fulcrum that represents the image plane. The "slice" thickness generally varies from 3–5 mm with linear machines the image layer may be narrower for multi- or pluridirectional units that travel through complex three-dimensional movements.

COMPUTED TOMOGRAPHY

CT with its two-dimensional and three-dimensional reconstruction capabilities is probably the most useful, unique and precise imaging modality for presurgical assessment. If multiple sites in the maxilla, mandible, or both are being evaluated or proposed, it may even be the most cost-effective technique. Plain tomographic imaging of multiple sites is quite labors, intensive, and thus the cost tend to be much higher than for one or two sites. In addition, most contemporary work stations and software used process the CT image data are rapid, detailed, and allow visualization of the proposed site on a 1:1 ratio, i.e. life-sized. Furthermore because the most appropriate approach to a successful implant is multidisciplinary, the assistance of a medical or oral and maxillofacial radiologist is appropriate because they also interpret, with greater expertise the tomographic and CT images for problems other than the implant assessment.

INTRATREATMENT EVALUATION

The use of radiography for intra treatment assessment of implants is:

1. To assess the integration status, the amount of "bone-fill" around the implant.
2. To assist the clinician in determining the optimum time for the second-stage procedure, if required. This evaluation is perhaps the most limited in term of radiographic technique.

Available to depict in any detail the extent of the osseointegration. A periapical radiograph can display only a small portion of the implant interface, usually seen as radiopaque "bone" adjacent to the V-shaped threads. And the technique is also very sensitive to positioning errors. This two-dimensional picture is very limited and the use of a radiograph alone would not be of much value. Clinical information about the implant status also must be evaluated.

Recently, attempts have been made to calculate the area of bone within the "triangle" of the thread as an objective measure of the amount of integration. Such quantification is very limited because the implant is round and the thread is circumferential. Perhaps the future use of CCD imagers with software developed to project a three-dimensional image of the implant and peri-implant bone will allow a more precise and detailed view of the integration of the bone about the implant and will assist the clinician in determining the appropriate time for the prosthetic phase of the implant.

POSTSURGICAL ASSESSMENT

As in the presurgical assessment of root form implant, several imaging technique are available for periodic evaluation. The use of tomography for longitudinal monitoring of prosthesis, however, is limited because of the time and expense as well as the inability of this technique to image the overall implant area. Similarly, CT probably is contraindicated because of the image artifact created by metals would obscure the information. This same artifact might be observed with root form implants. Consequently, current periodic radiographic follow-up can best be achieved by the use of intraoral and panoramic radiograph and potentially by electronic or solid-state detector.

13 Teleradiology for Dentistry

Rapid advances are occurring in telecommunications. These advances are having an important effect on the ways individuals and institutions communicate and do business. Funds are transferred almost instantaneously around the world via electronic networks. Credit is approved or denied internationally following the telecommunication of information encoded on the magnetic strip of credit card. The "fax" is replacing mail for the rapid transfer of written information. And access to computer network for data interchange is growing exponentially. Gilder describe this new age of "business built on sand and glass waves" as the "telecoms." He estimated that, in the next decade or so, microchip will contain a billion or more transistors, expanding a millionfold the cost effectiveness of computer hardware and making sophisticated "telecomputers" affordable for every household. Not surprisingly, these changes should have a great effect on the daily activities of dental practices.

HISTORICAL PERSPECTIVE

In 1774, George Lesage built a telegraph using one wire for each letter of the alphabet. Some 40 years later, Francis Ronalds demonstrated a single wire electrostatic telegraph. Teleprinting was not achieved before the late 1850s. Bell invented the telephone in 1875, which enabled the telegraphic lines to carry voice. Although the electronic transfer of radiograph was theoretically possible at the time Roentgen discovered X-radiation in1895, the long distance transmission of dental radiographs was probably first performed via telegraph in the 1920s. Success in this endeavor by the Western Union Telegraph Company was reported in 1920: "Even the filled root canals show up well. This service is available commercially should you wish to consult with a distant dentist." nevertheless, this service does not appear to have been of great success, perhaps because the idea was well ahead of the technology at the time, making such transmission impractical for general use.

Wenzel and Frovin suggested that the first practical transmission of a "roentgenographic facsimile" over a telephone line was performed in 1950 by scanning radiograph with light, then transmitting analog signals. The receiver was a photographic plate exposed to light in a pattern determined by the transmitted signal. The plate was then processed chemically. This was almost identical to the process earlier for telegraphic transmission.

Telemedicine developed with the use of television in the 1960s. Initially, analog systems were used, which were subject to transmission artifacts due to noise. Later digital systems were applied, using slow-scan television as the input device to digitize conventional film radiographs.

Radiologic informatics has developed rapidly in medicine during the past few years. Many systems are now commercially available for the transmission of radiographs in the form of Picture Archiving and Communicating Systems (PACS) and Image.

Transmission of dental radiographs also has potential value for forensic identification. Teeth are among the most resilient of human remains, and frequently, they carry unmistakable clues to the identity of a deceased person.

ADVANCES IN DENTAL IMAGE ACQUISITION

The need to scan or digitize traditional radiographs soon will become obsolete in density. Several direct systems are available for intraoral dental radiography using charge-coupled devices (CCDs).

In addition to the radiovisiography (RVG) system of trophy radiologie (Vincennes, France), which is now in its fourth generation, Gendex (Chicago) has produced an intraoral, direct digital system, the VIXA. Regam (Sweden) has a similar device named the "Sens-A-Ray," and Villa Sistemi Medicali (Buccinasco, Italy) sells the "Flash-Dent" system in many parts of the world. All four of these systems record the images in tagged image format file (TIFF). Thus, current telecommunication and image analysis software systems should be able to handle images from them all. In addition to facilitating teleradiology, these systems offer reduced patient exposure to radiation, and a wider range of contrast compared with conventional intraoral radiography. A range of image-processing enhancement procedures are also possible.

Prototype systems that use linear array CCDs have been developed by Dove and co-workers at the University of the University of Texa, San Antonio for both panoramic and cephalometric radiography. Extraoral indirect digital radiography is available using the Fuji CR (Fuji Corp, Odawara City, Japan). The computed radiography (CR) system uses a storage phosphor in place of film and processing is accomplished by laser scanning.

Similar systems are available from Vortech/Kodak (Rchester, NY). Others are being developed by Agfa (Antwerp, Begium) and Siemens (Bensheim, Germany).

APPROACHES TO TELECOMPUTING

Three broad approaches currently are used for telecomputing:

1. dedicated lines or private leased lines specifically for continuous access between sites.
2. switched (shared) telephone lines [generally using Integrated Systems Digital Networks (ISDN), or switch -56]
3. wideband electronic mail.

Dedicated and Switched Telephone Lines

A channel is defined as a path within a line through which information flows; whereas a line is the configured physical equipment for telecommunications. There are three types of channels: simplex, half-duplex, and full-duplex. Simplex channels only allow transmission in one direction and need to be used in loop configurations to allow feedback to the originating source. Half-duplex describes a two-way channel that only permits unidirectional transmissions at one time. This channel uses a two-wire format without frequency spectrum subdivision, and is the mode for present switched—telephone systems. Simultaneous receiving and transmission is possible with full-duplex channels, and these are ideal for rapid detection-and-correction of transmission errors. Dedicated lines are permanent circuits that only run between specified sites; whereas the switched-service opens to the full international telephone network (Fig. 13.1).

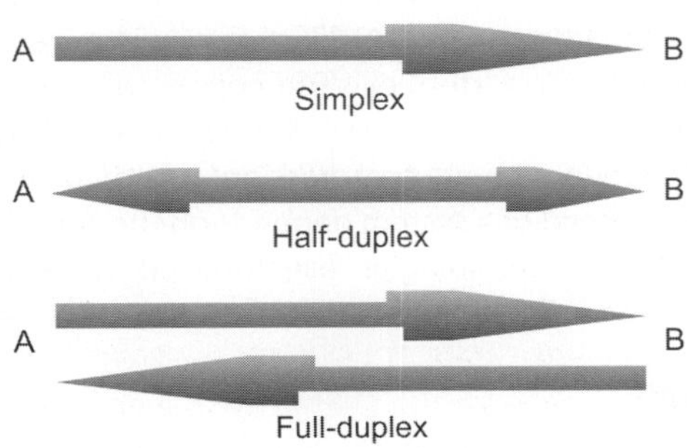

Fig. 13.1: Types of channels

Early telegram links carried up to about 30 words per minute or 15 bits per second. Now, most telephone cables carry many thousand voice channels, each with a capacity of 9600 bits per second. To transmit digital information using such voice lines, it is necessary for the data to be converted to a "voice", or modulated analog signal, via a modem at the transmitting end, and then to be reconverted to digital form through demodulation via a modem at the receiving end. This process is relatively slow for the transmission of the large number of bits of information that make up a digital image, and has a relatively high chance of bit error, estimated to reach as high as one error per 2000 bits transmitted. Using a standard 2400 baud modem, a 32-kbyte, third-generation RVG image would take about 2 minutes to transmit. Without compression, a fourth-generation,192-kbyte image of a single periapical area would take up to 12 minutes to transmit in one direction with voice-quality analog lines.

Through the digitization of existing telephone networks, the integration of existing and anticipated telecommunication services, the end-to-end sigaling, and the standardization of equipment and protocols, Integrating Systems Digital Networks (ISDN) aim to provide a single, efficient "bits pipe" and a single, standard "socket in the wall" for both voice and non-voice communication needs. Such systems will serve and connect all users around the globe. Throughout much of the world, data transmission standards are set by the International Telegraph and Telephone Consultative Committee (CCITT).

For leased lines, much larger "bit pipes" are available. These are necessary for the much larger image used in medicine. High-speed (wideband) transmission facilities are available from common carries at rates of 1.5 Mbit/sec (T1), 6.4 Mbit/sec (T2), 46 Mbit/sec (T3), 281 Mbit/sec (T4). Broadband ISDN (B-ISDN), using fiberoptic technology, is being developed that will allow transmissions between 150 Mbit/sec and 600 Mbit/sec. The big question is when such transmission rates become available on switched networks. AT&T currently is experimenting with computed systems to "smarten" existing copper wire circuits to permit transmission rates of 90–150 Mbit/sec. At 90 Mbit/sec, it will be possible to transmit true video without compression. It should be remembered, however, that the speed of a system depends on the slowest component. Current image storage technologies may not support transmission much beyond 6 Mbit/sec.

Electronic-mail

Packet-switched networks initially were developed in the late 1960s in an attempt to achieve effective sharing of computer resources. These networks have developed into the Internet is a worldwide collection of thousands of interconnected computer networks used by more than one million persons daily. Either the Transmission Control Protocol/Internet Protocol (TCP/IP) or the Open Systems Interconnection (OSI) is used, and gateways exit that translate between these two protocols. Since its creation, the Internet has grown exponentially in terms of the number of networks connected to it.

Toward the Future

The specific goal of ongoing teleradiology research for dentistry should be directed toward finding and testing cost-effective and efficient methods that are practical for use in general dental offices. Systems need to be evaluated in terms of transmission speed, image quality, cost, convenience, and confidentiality.

Transmission Time

Using Switch-56, images of 32 kbytes can be transferred both transcontinentally and intercontinentally in 4.6 seconds. It is possible to take a radiograph in real time in <1 second, store it in the computer in a few moments, and have the image ready for transfer in about 20 seconds. Hence, the total time from exposure to reception at a remote site need to be no more than 30 seconds to 1 minute, provided that the switched line is not busy.

Image translation initially took 10 minutes, but has been reduced to 10 seconds. Transmission speeds vary with the traffic in the system. Unlike ISDN, however, it is not necessary for the recipient to be on-line to receive the image. Transferred files are stored in a loco-regional mainframe computer to be accessed at the convenience of the recipient if FTP is used. With TELNET, it is possible for the recipient to control the sender's computer to choose the files to be retrieved.

Image Quality

Digital subtraction of transmitted and unaltered, received images has shown that there is no loss of image detail, using both switched—digital telephone lines and electronic-mail systems. Images altered by gradient enhancements performed by the recipient can be returned to their original state prior to subtraction by remapping the gray levels. The darkest pixels were reassigned as black and the lightest as white, with linear rescaling in between.

Confidentiality

Confidentiality is always a concern with personal data, especially information related to health. It is theoretically possible for recipients to forward as many copies to as many sites as they wish; however, this is no different than silver halide films that can be copied using duplicating film. Encryption certainly needs careful consideration as dentistry moves forward into the age of electronics (Figs 13.2 and 13.3).

Cost

ISDN/Switch-56 is currently quite expensive in the United States when viewed from the perspective of a general dental practice. The cost will probably decline rapidly, however, in the immediate future.

Membership in Internet can be quite expensive for institutions; however, commercially available access, usually using local telephone connections is available at cheaper rate.

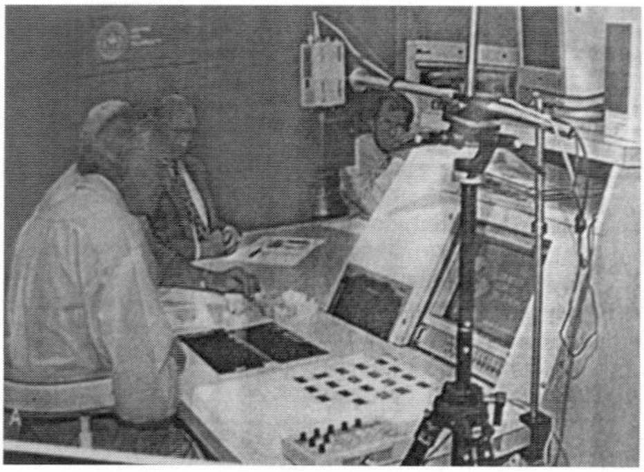

Fig. 13.2: Consulting specialist at the transmission and receiving console

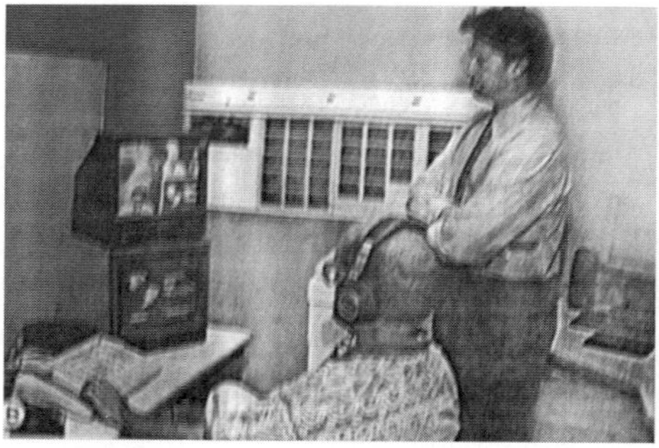

Fig. 13.3: Technical staff monitoring the transmission system

Convenience

Provided both sites are on-line, ISDN/Switch-56 is convenient to use. Electronic mail systems, however, provide the convenience to the recipient of being able to open the transmitted files at leisure (FTP) or to select files to be transmitted from a remote site. This is particularly convenient when a difference in time zones is a factor.

14 Photostimulable Phosphor Radiography

Film-based radiography remains the most commonly used imaging method. New imaging modalities such as computed tomography (CT), magnetic resonance (MR) imaging, ultrasonography, and positron-emission tomography (PET) are driving radiology toward digital image interpretation and diagnosis. A new radiographic digital imaging technology, photostimulable phosphor radiography (PPR) has potential to improve dental radiography and is likely to become increasingly common over the next 5 years. In 1947 it was proposed that if a phosphor were energized by exposure to X-rays, a latent image could be produced and stimulated at a later time with infrared light. Commercialization of these methods was first publicly presented in 1981 at the International Congress of Radiology, and the first technical paper describing this methodology was published in 1983. Since then, there have been numerous improvements in phosphors and imaging systems.

The technique is variously referred to as PPR, digital luminescence radiography, storage phosphor radiography, computed radiography and radioluminography.

PRINCIPLES OF PHOTOSTIMULABLE PHOSPHOR RADIOGRAPHY

Several attributes are required of a storage phosphor material. First, the compound must create and store the latent image without appreciable degradation until it is ready to be scanned. Second, it must be possible to stimulate efficiently the phosphor with light so that the stored energy in the latent image can be released. Third, the released energy must have a wavelength that can be readily detected in the presence of the stimulating light.

Europium-doped barium fluorohalide [(Ba, Eu) FX, where X is Br, Cl or I] is the most commonly used compound. Europium is added as an impurity, acting as an activator to create luminescence centers (holes). The storage phosphor is covered with a protective coating, which helps prevent physical and atmospheric damage to the storage phosphor. This combination of storage phosphor, base, and protective coating is referred to as a storage-phosphor plate.

When the storage phosphor is exposed to X-rays, an electron of the Eu^{+2} ion is excited to the conduction band, creating an electron vacancy (hole) at the trivalent europium site (Eu^{+3}). This electron is then trapped at a halogen vacancy (F-center) in the crystalline lattice of the storage phosphor. About half of the holes and trapped electrons recombine spontaneously and cause luminescence. The other half form metastable states, the local concentration of holes and trapped electrons being proportional to the local X-ray exposure. Because latent image formation is efficient and the phosphor absorbs much more of the radiation than non-screen film, much lower exposures are required than for non-screen dental film; however, random thermal processes because an exponential decay of the latent image through phosphorescence, with approximately 25–50% of the stored signal being lost within 1 hour after exposure. The remainder of the latent image persists for periods of days.

Because film serves as the X-ray detector and as the display medium, careful attention has to be paid to X-ray exposure to obtain optimal images. With storage phosphor systems, image acquisition and display are separate events; plus, storage phosphors have linear responses to X-ray exposure. It is possible to underexpose or overexpose storage phosphors and still produce clinically acceptable images with standard image processing techniques. With film, exposure adjustments are required to compensate for variations among subjects and among anatomic areas imaged. With storage phosphors, even if improper exposure techniques are used, the final image can be optimized with software. With most storage-phosphor systems, the intent is to make the digital images resemble, as nearly as possible, film-based images.

Although storage phosphors are readable for many days, it is best to read them as soon as possible. A significant fraction of the decay occurs within the first few minutes after exposure. Although the decay is usually not clinically important, it could be a factor if image feature densities (i.e. of oral hard tissues) were to be quantified.

Once the storage phosphor is read, it is flooded with light (often high intensity) to erase any remaining image and to prepare the storage phosphor for the next exposure. Because the latent image is erased by exposure to light, care should be used to avoid exposing the storage phosphor to excessive amounts of background light (including darkroom light). After exposure, the background radiation can expose the phosphor. If the plate has not been used within 24 hours, it is good policy to erase it again before use (Figs 14.1 to 14.3).

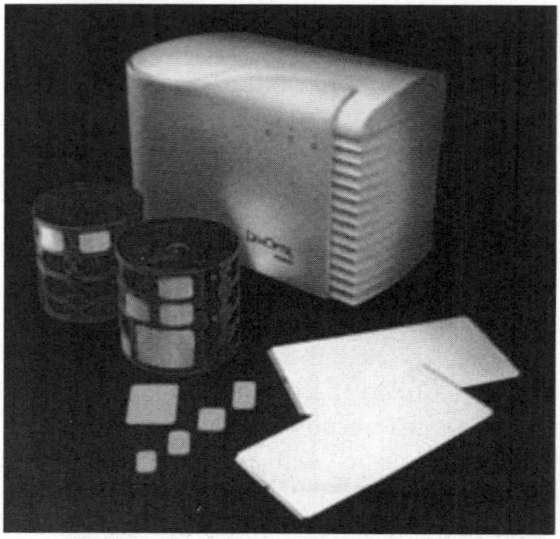

Fig. 14.1: The DenOptix processing unit

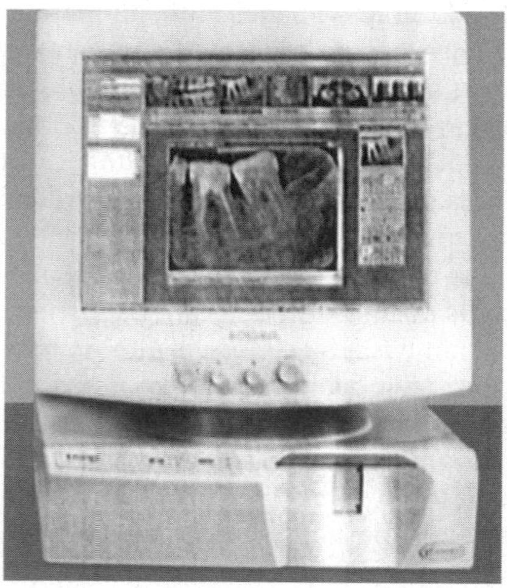

Fig. 14.2: Digora FMX system

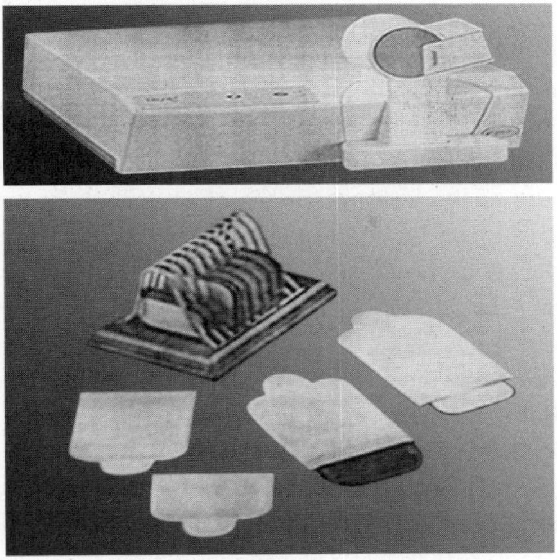

Fig. 14.3: Soredex imaging plate Autoloader for use with the Digora FMX system and Digora imaging plates

Although phosphors are stable through time, the plates can be damaged; modest caution should be exercised when handling the plates. Because accumulations of dirt on the storage-phosphor plate can compromise image quality, the plates should be periodically cleaned with a screen cleaner.

The storage phosphor based images can be displayed on cathode ray tube (CRT) monitors or printed. Monitors and the associated workstations vary a great deal with regard to quality and available software for image processing.

The digital signal of a PPR image can be stored or transferred over network or telephone lines to other sites or to digital storage devices; PPR systems can be made compliant to Digital Communications in Medicine (DICOM) so that they can be interfaced to existing and future picture archiving and communications systems (PACS).

Actual and Potential Advantages of Photostimulable Phosphor Radiography

Actual and potential advantages of PPR are as follows:

1. Storage phosphor plates can be reused indefinitely.
2. PPR can be used with existing X-ray sources.

3. Linear or logarithmic response to radiation is available. A feature of interest in a dental image may appear in a radio dense area and be imaged in the toe area of the characteristic curve of film. Conversely a feature may appear in a radiolucent area. In either case, the feature is shown with reduced contrast and may be difficult or impossible to see. Because of the linear response of phosphors to radiation, such features can often be seen by subjecting the image to electronic image processing. The linear response may also prove to be particularly important in studied in which the intent is to quantify small changes in oral hard tissues.
4. There is wide exposure range and fewer retakes. Compared with dental film, PPR is much more lenient with regard to using a specific exposure for a particular film type and patient. What would be an underexposed or overexposed image with film may appear as a normal PPR image.
5. Less radiation is required for most diagnostic tasks. For some diagnostic tasks, PPR require 90% less X-ray exposure time than film.
6. No chemical processing is required (chemicals are allergenic and potential pollutants).
7. Image processing of acquired images (post-processing) is available. Because PPR images are digital, they can be processed to enhance features of interest and to suppress interfering anatomic structures and noise. At the simplest level, magnification may enhance visibility of features considerably.
8. Images can be transferred to other sites. Because the PPR images are in digital form, they can be transferred to consultants or third party carriers at local or remote area.
9. Images can be easily and inexpensively stored and retrieved. A great advantage of digital images over film based images is that they can be easily stored and retrieved. Such storage and retrieval systems are already cost-competitive with film based systems. With marketplace competition and improved technology; these costs should continue to decline.
10. Computer-aided diagnosis. With digital images, there exists the possibility for developing computer programs to aid the practitioner in making diagnosis. Current efforts along these lines have been mostly focused on caries.

Disadvantages of Photostimulable Phosphor Radiography

1. It would seem that the initial cost of a PPR system would be recovered in time because of the diminished number of retakes, elimination of chemical processing, and reduced cost for image storage and retrieval. To date, however, cost-benefit studies of PPR systems in dentistry have not been published.
2. The spatial resolution of film exceeds that of PPR. It is not clear, however, that the increased spatial resolution available with film results in improved diagnosis. This area needs additional research attention.
3. In general, currently available image processing routines have not been optimized for dental diagnostic tasks and may not have reached their potential. It is also not clear which of the available image processing routines improve diagnosis. Some of the routines are time intensive and may increase the time required to make diagnosis without improving diagnostic success rates.
4. Although PPR image display is much more flexible than film image display, the display method still may not be optimal. Additional research is needed to determine the requirements for image display in dentistry.
5. Images may initially appear different from film based images. Although manufacturer's attempt, through image processing, to provide images that are similar in appearance to the film based images, it may take a while for the clinician to become comfortable with PPR images and image processing in general.
6. Phosphor plates must be packaged in sterile envelopes.

15 Ultrasonic Imaging Technique (Ultrasound)

Ultrasound is noninvasive, nonionizing imaging technique. Ultrasonography or ultrasound uses sound as sonar does to image structures deep within soft tissue. Ultrasonic scanners use a transducer to convert electrical energy into high frequency sound waves that pass into the tissue. As the waves strike tissues of different densities, some of the vibrational energy is reflected back to the scanning transducer, where the sound waves are converted back to electrical energy. This electrical energy is amplified, enhanced, and displayed on a video monitor.

Nowadays ultrasound systems have more than one mode of scanning and can demonstrate "real time" imaging of physiologic motion. Ultrasound (US) is particularly good when adjacent structures transmit sound at significantly different rates, such as between a sialolith and surrounding soft tissue. It is also good at determining the outlines of structures but not necessarily their contents. US is inexpensive, and produces no side effects.

Doppler US is particularly useful in identifying soft tissue vascular lesions. Doppler uses the fact that moving red blood cells shift the reflected vibrational energy in proportion to the velocity of the blood.

Ultrasound is sensitive technique, and an experienced specialist is needed to develop and interpret a good ultrasound image.

PRINCIPLE

The phenomenon perceived as sound is the result of periodic changes in the pressure of air against the ear-drum. The periodicity of these changes lies anywhere between 1500 and 20,000 cycles per second (Hz). By definition, ultrasound has a periodicity of greater than 20 kHz. Thus, it is distinguished from other mechanical waveforms simply by having a vibratory frequency greater than the audible range. Diagnostic ultrasonography, the clinical application of ultrasound, employs vibratory frequencies in the range of 1–20 MHz.

SONOGRAPHIC SYSTEM AND TECHNIQUE

Scanners used for sonography generate electrical impulses that are converted into ultra-high frequency sound waves by a transducer, which is simply a device that can convert one form of energy into another, in this case electrical energy into sonic energy.

The most important component of the transducer is a thin piezoelectric crystal or material made up of a great number of dipoles arranged in a geometric pattern. A dipole may be thought of as a distorted molecule that appears to have a positive charge on one end and a negative charge on the other. Currently the most widely used piezoelectric material is lead zirconate titanate (PZT). The electrical impulse generated by the scanner causes the dipoles within the crystal to realign themselves with the electrical field and thus suddenly change the crystals thickness. This abrupt change begins a series of vibrations that produce the sound waves that are transmitted into the tissues being examined.

As the ultrasonic beam passes through, or interacts with, tissues of different acoustic impedance, it is attenuated by a combination of absorption, reflection, refraction and diffusion. Sonic waves that are reflected back (echoes) toward the transducer cause a change in the thickness of the piezoelectric crystal, which in turn produces an electrical signal that is amplified, processed and ultimately displayed on a monitor. In this system, the transducer serves as both a transmitter and a receiver. High-resolution ultrasonography systems operating in the B-mode, which produces a picture of a slice of tissue, may achieve an axial (depth) resolution of 0.5 mm or less and a lateral resolution of 1mm or less. Techniques currently in use permit echoes to be processed at a sufficiently rapid rate to allow for the perception of motion. This is referred to as real-time imaging.

There are different US display modes:

A-mode - Amplitude mode
B-mode - Brightness mode
M-mode - Motion mode
Real time

In *A-mode*, echoes are displayed as peaks or spikes projecting from a baseline. The baseline identifies the central axes of the beam. Spike height is proportional to echo density, i.e. strong echoes producing large spikes (Fig. 15.1).

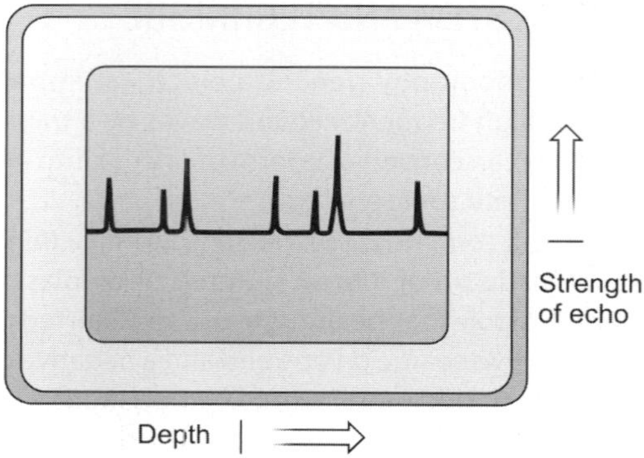

Fig. 15.1: A-mode, echoes are displayed as peaks or spikes projecting from a baseline

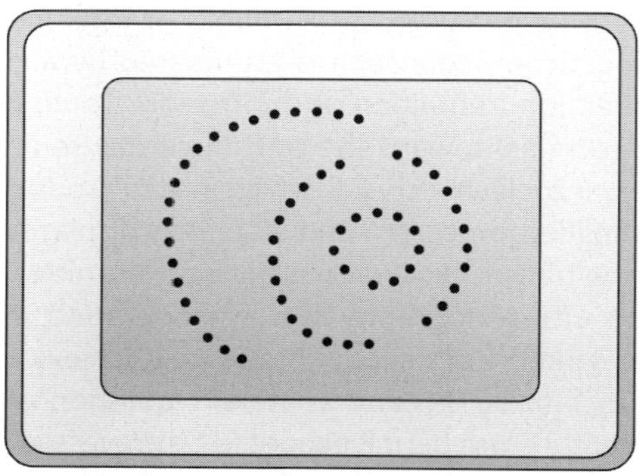

Fig. 15.2: B-mode, echoes are displayed as dots

B-mode: Produce a picture of slice of tissue. Mainly in abdominal. Echoes are displayed as dots (Fig. 15.2). The images are two dimensional If multiple B-mode images are watched in rapid sequence, they become real time images.

M-mode: It is another way of displaying motion and is shown as a function of time. Result is wavy line. This mode is commonly used for cardiac ultrasound, the movement of a part of a body such as a fetal heart (Fig. 15.3).

Real time: This mode displays motion by showing the images of the part of the body under the transducer as it is being scanned. The image change with each movement of the transducer or if any part of the body is moving.

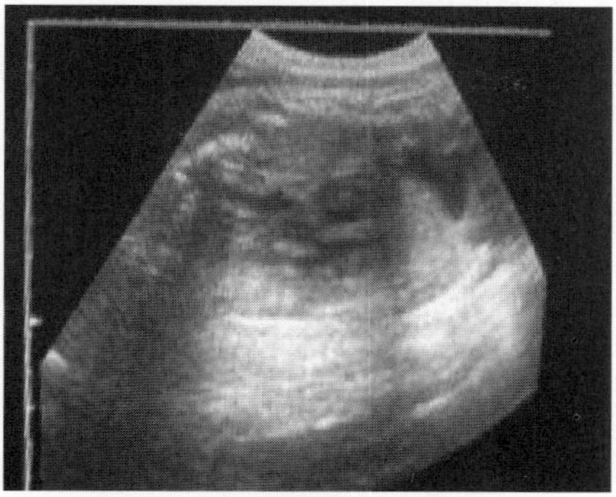

Fig. 15.3: M-mode, commonly used for cardiac ultrasound, the movement of a part of a body such as a fetal heart

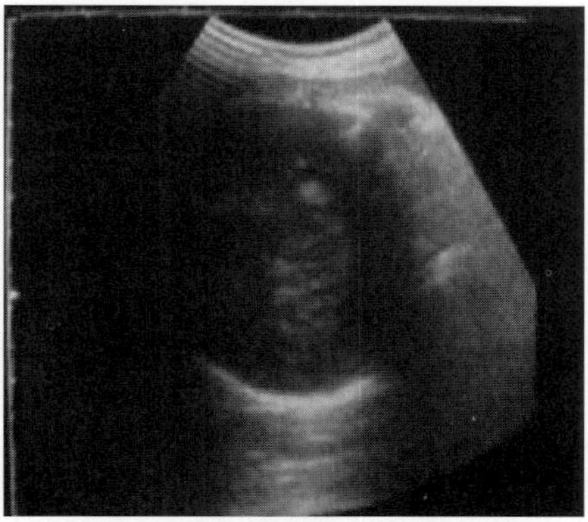

Fig. 15.4: Real time image, it is possible to freeze the display images, holding it stationary so that it can be studied or measured

The movements are shown on the monitor in real time as it occurs. In most real time units it is possible to freeze the display images, holding it stationary so that it can be studied or measured. It produces 10 images/second (Fig. 15.4).

In radiography, image is produced by transmitted radiation, in sonography the image is produced by the reflected portion of the beam. The fraction of the beam that is reflected back to the transducer is dependent on the acoustic impedance of the tissue, which is a product of its density (and thus the velocity of sound through it) and the beam's angle of incidence. Because of its acoustic impedance a tissue has an internal echo pattern that is characteristic. Consequently, not only can changes in

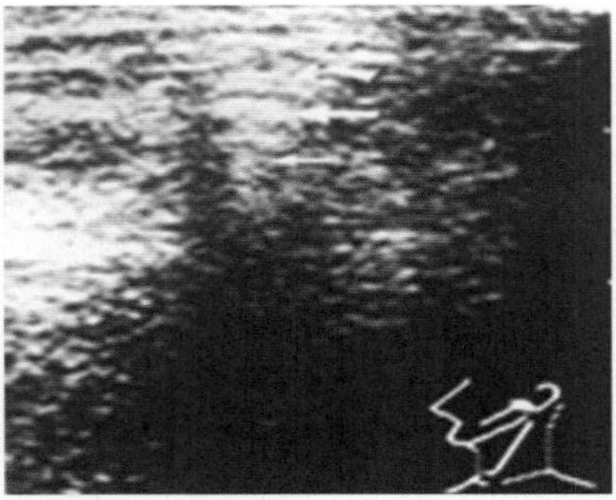

Fig. 15.5: Ultrasound image of the TMJ. In closed-mouth position

echo patterns delineate different tissues, they may also be correlated with pathologic changes in a tissue. The interpretation of sonograms, then, relies on knowledge of both the physical properties of ultrasound and the anatomy of tissues being scanned (Fig. 15.5).

BASIC RULES OF SCANNING

1. *Orientation of the image*: It is essential before scanning to check visually that side of the transducer produces which side of the image. This is done by putting a finger at one end of transducer and see where it appears on the screen. If incorrect rotate the transducer 1800 and check again. There is an indication for same, on the transducer (Fig. 15.6).
2. *Contact with patients skin*: The transducer must be moved across the patient's skin. Patients skin must be covered with coupling agent to prevent air trapped between skin and transducer as the air will form a barrier that reflect almost all the US waves, preventing them from penetrating the patient (Fig. 15.7).
   To obtain a good image a fluid medium is needed. This fluid is called as an acoustic coupling agent or gel. Water is not good coupling agent because it evaporates rapidly owing to the heat of the body. It also runs away over the patient's skin as the transducer is moved. The best coupling agent is water soluble gel.

Carbomer	–	10.0 g
EDTA	–	25 g
Propyl glycol	–	75.0 g
Trolamin	–	12.5 g
Distilled water	–	Upto 500 g

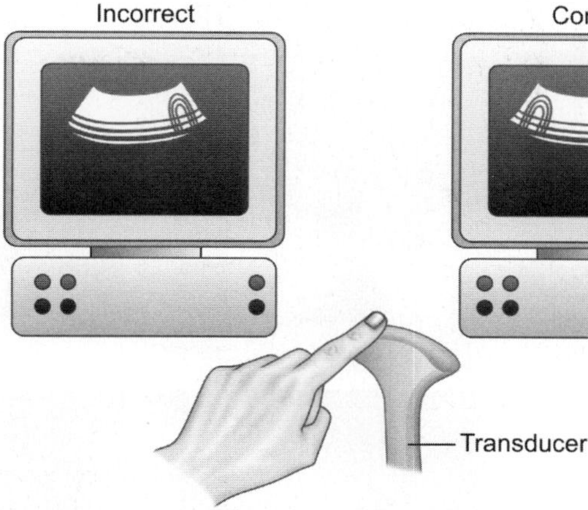

Fig. 15.6: Position of the transducer

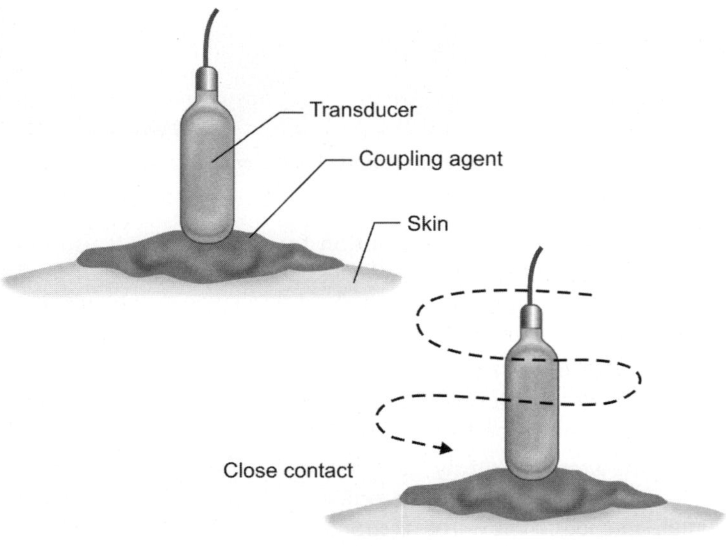

Fig. 15.7: Relation of the transducer with skin during imaging

3. *Background of the Image (Fig. 15.8)*:
   - ❑ White background with black echoes
   - ❑ Black background with white echoes
   - ❑ There is a switch to make this change.

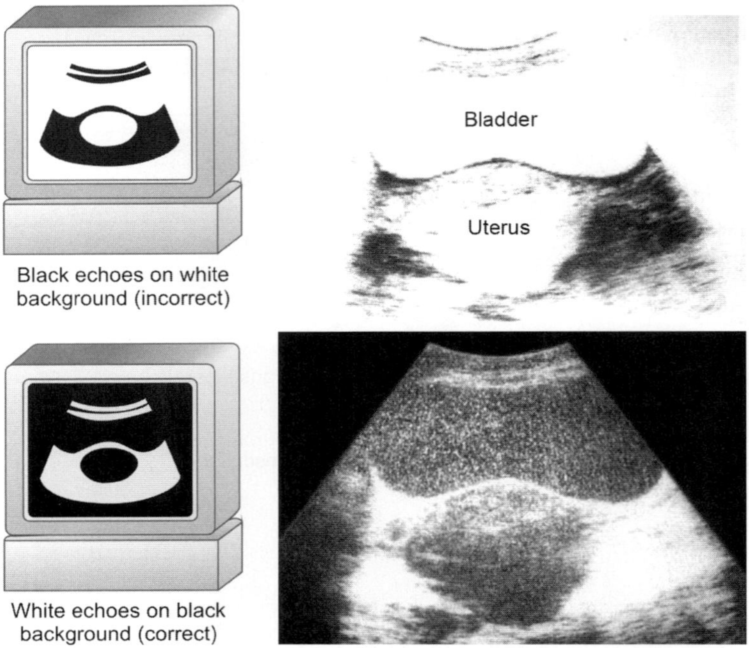

Fig. 15.8: Background of the image

4. *Frequency and resolution*:
   Higher frequency: Better resolution for smaller details use higher frequency but penetration will be less at higher frequency. Therefore, scanning is a compromise and highest frequency that is sufficient to penetrate deeply enough should be used.
5. *Focus the US beam*: As the part of interest will be at different depths, the focus of transducer should be adjusted accordingly or suitable transducer should be selected (Fig. 15.9).
6. *Gain*: The wrong sensitivity (gain) setting can make diagnosis inaccurate or even impossible. If the gain is too low, a solid may appear cystic without internal echoes. There will be no strong backwall effect (no enhancement).

   If the gain is too high—a fluid filled structure may fill with echoes and resemble a solid mass, for example, A cyst usually appears an echo free area and the structure behind the cyst is enhanced. There are no echoes from within the cyst as there are no impedance interfaces within the liquid. The echoes behind the cyst are over compensated and appear enhanced called as 'strong back wall effect' (Fig. 15.10).

   If there are echoes within a cyst, these may be real or art factual.

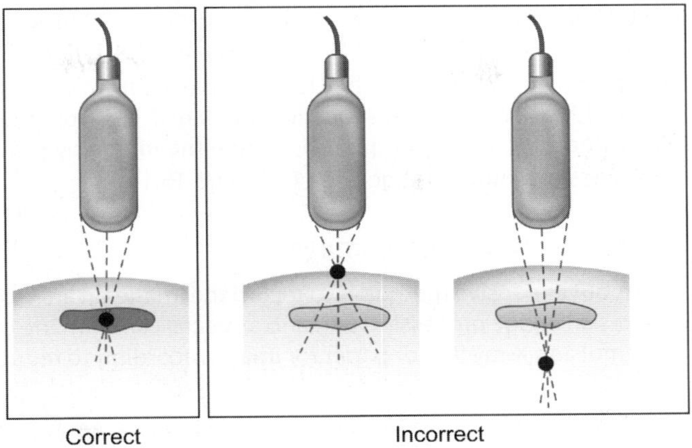

Fig. 15.9: Focus of transducer

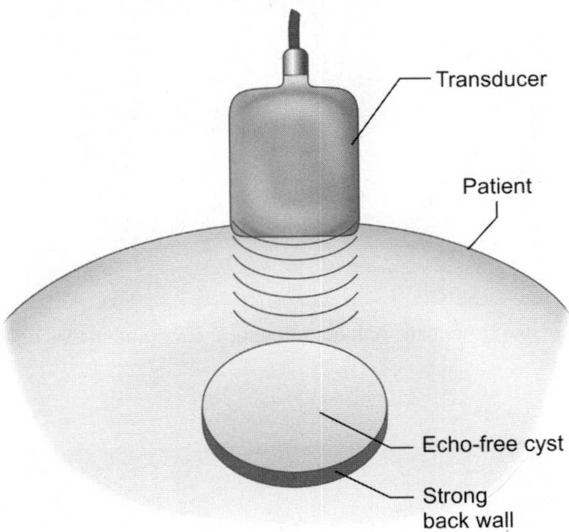

Fig. 15.10: The echoes behind the cyst are over compensated and appear enhanced called as 'strong back wall effect'

7. *Acoustic enhancement and shadowing*: Clear liquids allow US to pass directly through without much alteration, so that the echoes that come from tissue from behind liquid are usually enhanced (brighter). This is known as acoustic enhancement.

   Dense materials such as bones or calculi cast shadows on structure behind them, the US waves do not go through them. This is known as acoustic shadowing.

8. Use multiple projections at different angles to confirm any suspected abnormality to avoid artifact (Figs 15.11 and 15.12).
9. *Reverberation*: It occurs when the US beam passes from one tissue to another with a very different acoustic impedance, e.g. from intestinal gas to liver or ribs. It can completely change the image by producing parallel lines or a mirror image (Figs 15.13 and 15.14).

Permanent Recording of the Image

1. The best but expensive method is to record the image on an X-ray film. It requires an image processing unit and a special camera. One can use single emulsion X-ray film or paper for image recording to reduce cost (Fig. 15.15).

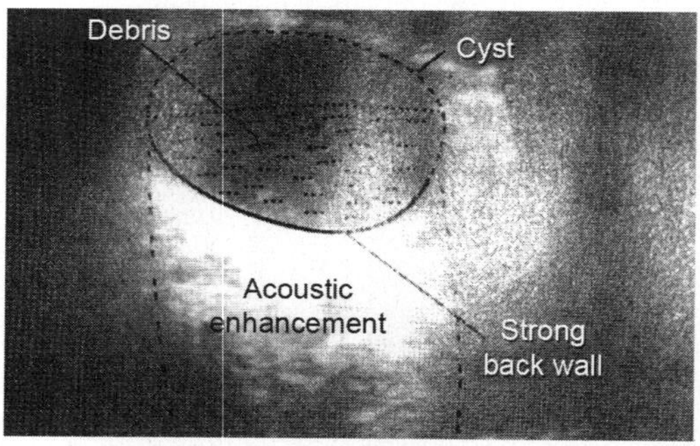

Fig. 15.11: Acoustic enhancement and strong back wall effect

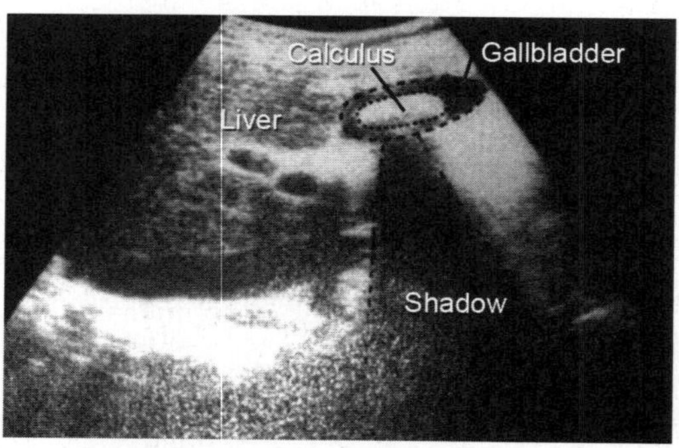

Fig. 15.12: Acoustic enhancement and shadowing

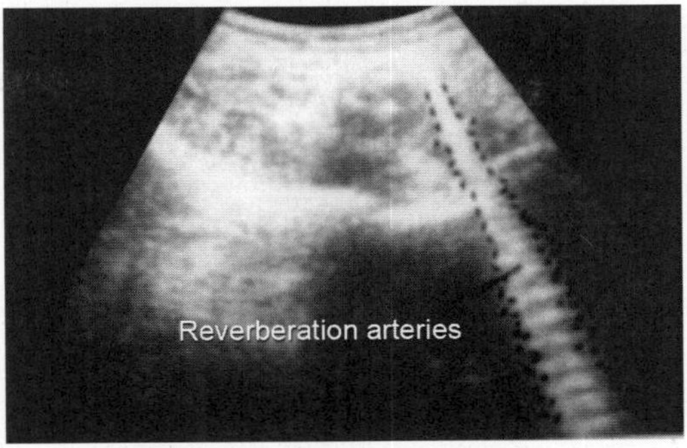

Fig. 15.13: Reverberation, it occurs when the US beam passes from one tissue to another with a very different acoustic impedance producing parallel lines

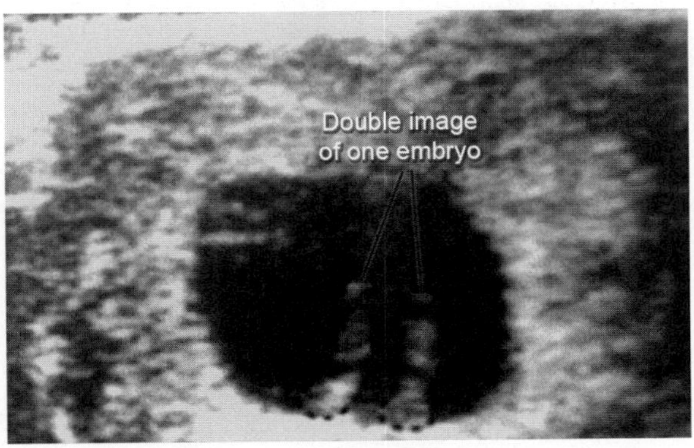

Fig. 15.14: Reverberation, it occurs when the US beam passes from one tissue to another with a very different acoustic impedance producing a mirror image

2. There is (1) special self-processing camera and (2) Special films—attached to the US unit which record the image.
3. There is an image recording or printer prints are obtained on special glossy paper. The images are satisfactory.
4. The image on screen can be photographed on black and white film by using reflex cameras. The film is then processed and printed in usual way (Fig. 15.16).
5. All the relevant measurement, findings are recorded in patients record at the time of scan (Fig. 15.17).

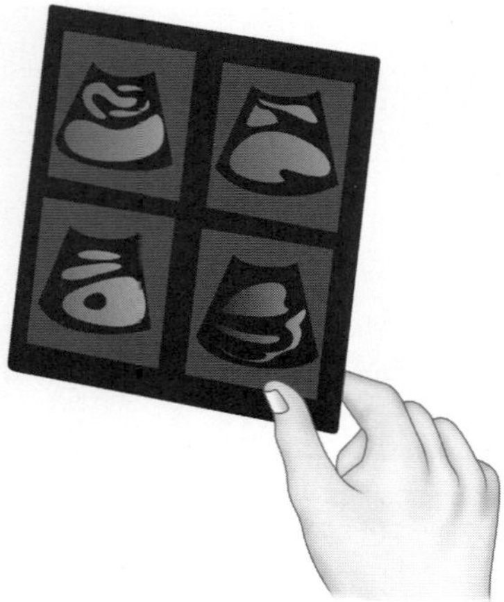

Fig. 15.15: USG images on an X-ray film

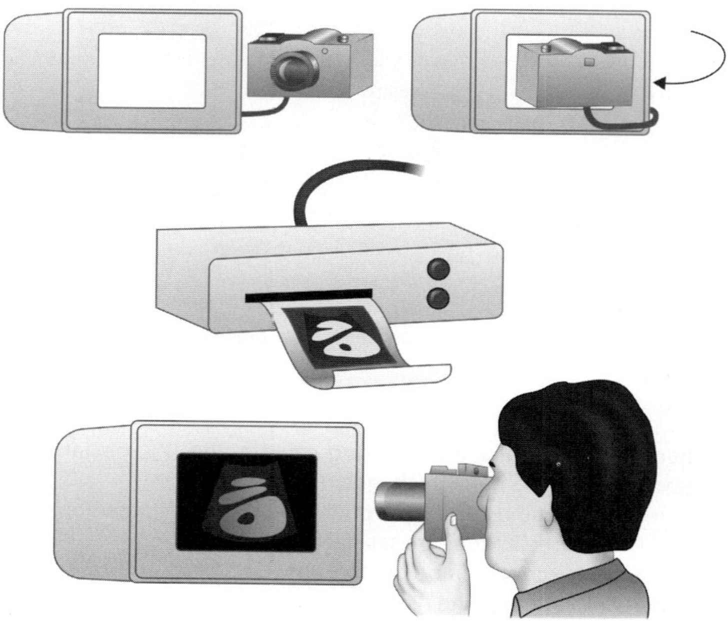

Fig. 15.16: The image on screen can be photographed on black and white film by using reflex cameras. The film is then processed and printed in usual way

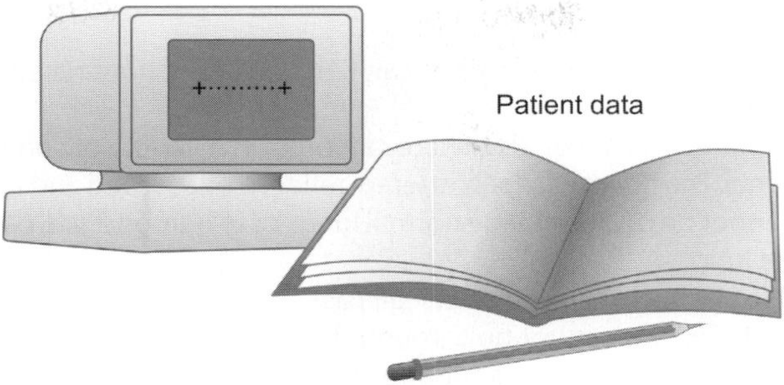

Fig. 15.17: The patients record at the time of scan

Dental Applications of Ultrasonography

1. In the region of the head and neck diagnostic ultrasound has been applied to the evaluation of many structures and conditions: lymph nodes, post surgical edema and hematoma, and the eye, thyroid gland, and parotid, submandibular, and sublingual salivary glands.
2. To demonstrate the thickness of the masticatory mucosa, it is also useful for determining the extent of soft tissue displacement under dentures by the forces of occlusion.
3. Ultrasonography should be the initial imaging study used for the examination of salivary gland lesions in children; most of such lesions are benign and are shown up clearly by sonography. In most cases, this technique permits differentiation of intraglandular and extraglandular lesions. Vascular lesion can be demonstrated more clearly through the use of color Doppler imaging.
4. Ultrasonography is the first line diagnostic procedure in the clarification of pathologic lesions of the major salivary gland because of lack of radiation exposure, there is free choice of echographic plane.
5. Ultrasound is helpful in ultrasound guided needle localization in the removal of multiple objects from soft tissue in the head and neck.
6. Ultrasound guided aspiration (fine needle aspiration).

Advantages of Ultrasound

1. Ionizing radiation is not used.
2. Provides good imaging of superficial masses.
3. Excellent for differentiating between solid and cystic masses.
4. Different echo signals are from different tumors.
5. Can be repeated as often as desired.

Disadvantages of Ultrasound

1. US cannot be used for gas filled cavities, and dense materials like bone. e.g. MA, skull, etc.
   Gas in the bowel or elsewhere can present a variety of sonographic patterns. The beam can be scattered, reflected, absorbed and refracted. US cannot be used to image normal lungs or to demonstrate pathology in the lung.
   Material such as bone or calculi cast shadows or structures behind them. US waves cannot go through them.
2. Significant subcutaneous fat and muscle can scatter US making the image of deeper structures less distinct. Sometimes muscle cause double image giving false impression of separation.
3. US is of limited value in diagnosis of inflammatory and obstructive diseases of salivary gland.
4. In salivary gland imaging, US produce no information about architecture
5. In head and neck its use is limited.
6. Dressing over wounds and drainage bags may cause contact problems.
7. Technique is operator dependant.

Advances in Ultrasound

1. Doppler US
2. Color Doppler US
3. Duplex Doppler US
4. Use of contrast agent in diagnostic US
5. US guided intervention
6. Power Doppler
7. ECHO
8. US biomicroscopy
9. Hybrid arrays
10. Elastography
11. Therapeutic US.

Doppler US

The Doppler effect is a change in the perceived frequency of sound emitted by a moving source. This effect was first described by Christian Doppler in 1843.

For example, an ambulance is moving 27 m/sec is blowing its siren at a frequency of 1000 Hz. The frequency ahead of siren is 1086 Hz while the frequency behind it is 926 Hz. A pedestrian would hear a frequency shift of 160 Hz. The only person hearing the true frequency of 1000 Hz would be the passenger in the vehicle (Fig. 15.18).

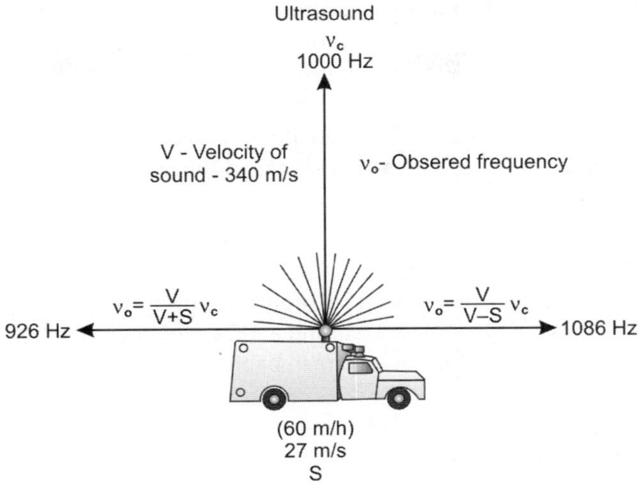

Fig. 15.18: Doppler ultrasound: The Doppler effect is a change in the perceived frequency of sound emitted by a moving source

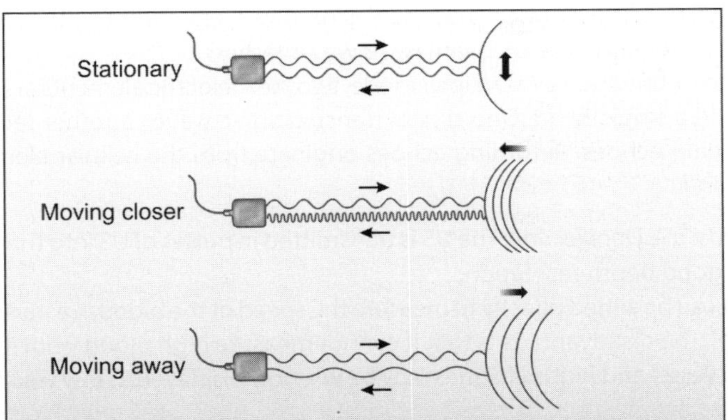

The difference between the transmitted and received frequencies is proportional to the speed with which the reflector is moving away from or approaching the transmitter. This phenomenon is called the Doppler effect and the difference between the frequencies is called the Doppler shift.

Fig. 15.19: Doppler effects of moving objects

When US is transmitted toward a stationary reflector, the reflected wave's echoes will be of same frequency as those originally transmitted.

If the reflector is moving toward the transmitter then the reflected frequency will be higher than the transmitted frequency (Fig. 15.19).

If the reflector is moving away from the transmitter, the reflected frequency will be lower than the transmitted frequency.

The difference between the transmitted and received frequencies is proportional to the speed with which the reflector is moving away from or approaching the transmitter. The phenomenon is called as Doppler Effect. The difference between frequencies is called the Doppler shift. In blood the moving reflectors are RBCs.

Indication of Doppler US

1. To detect and measure the rate of movement of any fluid such as blood.
2. Assessment of blood flow in carotid and carotid body tumors.
3. Assessment of ventricular system in babies by imaging through open fontanelles.
4. Volume of blood in blood vessel.
5. Obstruction in the blood vessel—thrombi, plug.

Two types of doppler US units

Continuous wave Doppler unit: The US is continuous and the unit measures high velocities accurately, but there is no depth resolution so that all the movement along the US beam is shown together.

In continuous wave Doppler mode, two piezoelectric elements are used both in a single head. One crystal transmit sonic waves another receives returning echoes. Returning echoes originate from the cellular elements of blood.

Pulsed wave Doppler unit: The US is transmitted in pulses of US into the body with good depth resolution.

It can be aimed directly to measure the speed of the blood in a particular vessel. The disadvantage is that it cannot measure high blood velocities in deep vessel and high velocities may be wrongly displayed as low velocities.

Color Doppler Ultrasound

The distribution and direction of flowing blood are shown as a two-dimensional image in which velocities are distinguished by different colors.

Two colors—**Red** denotes the flow/reflector is coming toward
Blue denotes the flow is moving away (Fig. 15. 20).

Advantages of Color Doppler

1. Arteries can be distinguished from vein.
2. Vessels too small can be seen.
3. Differentiation between vascular and non-vascular stage is simplified.

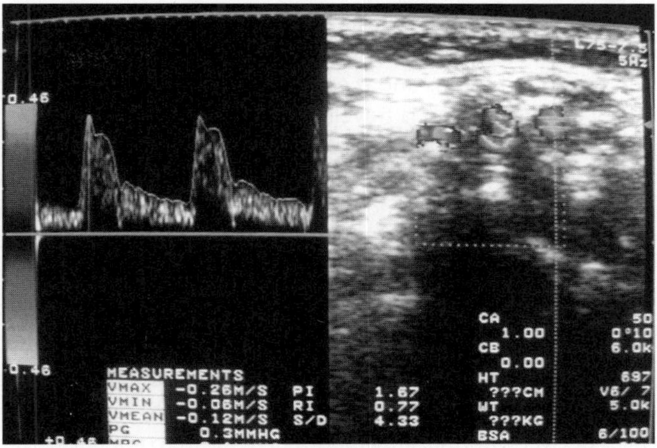

Fig. 15.20: Color Doppler: Red denotes the flow/reflector is coming toward. Blue denotes the flow is moving away

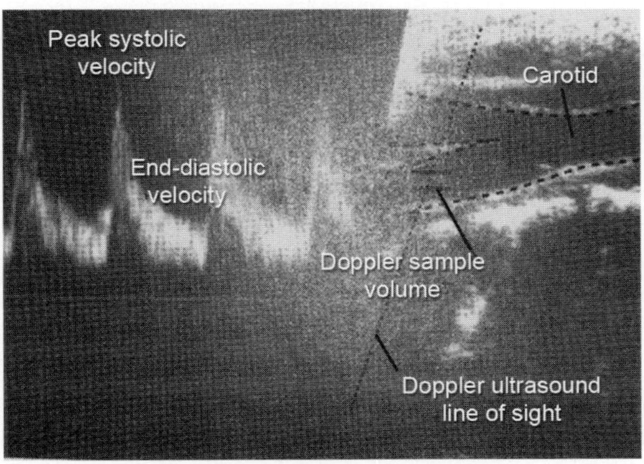

Fig. 15.21: Duplex Doppler US. Blood vessel is located by B-mode ultrasound imaging and then blood flow is measured by Doppler US

4. Visualization of flow throughout the entire lumen and facilitates detection of small intraluminal filling defects, e.g. small arterial plugs, thrombi.

Duplex Doppler US: Blood vessel is located by B-mode ultrasound imaging and then blood flow is measured by Doppler US. This combination of B-mode and Doppler system allows the reflector beam to be directed more accurately at any particular blood vessel (Fig. 15.21).

Power Doppler

The intensity of Doppler signal depends upon the volume of blood reflecting the sound pulses and the amplitude of the signal depends on the velocity at which blood is traveling. Small volumes of blood moving slowly produce a weak signal. This is difficult to define. One way to improve this situation is to integrate the energy from all the shift information in both directions together, thus increasing the overall power of the Doppler information and sensitivity of the system but at the expense of losing directional and velocity information.

It is sensitive in detecting blood flow in smaller vessels and vessels with slow flow.

Contrast agents in Diagnostic US: Intravenous ultrasound contrast agents are substances introduced into the vascular system to enhance contrast differences between normal and abnormal tissue or to enhance arterial or venous Doppler signal.

Two basic types of UCA's are available

1. Nonencapsulated air bubbles
2. Encapsulated air bubbles

The major goal of IV contrast agent is to increase the signal returning to the US transducer. The mechanism for signal enhancement is micro bubble back scatter which related to differences in microbubble versus blood compressibility. The net effect is increase in echogenicity. Increase echogenicity may be seen as increase in color or spectral Doppler signal strength or gray scale image intensity.

Another major effect of ultrasound contrast agents is enhancement of color, power and spectral Doppler. The application of UCAS to improve Doppler imaging in termed Doppler rescue.

Other potential uses for intravenous US contrast agents under current investigation include detecting and differentiating malignant from benign neoplasm in the breast and prostate and detecting abdominal hemorrhage.

Another novel application relates to tumor specific chemotherapy. This technique consists of IV injection of chemotherapeutic agent that contains microbubbles. Once the microbubbles reach the tumor, they are destroyed by a high power ultrasound signal and the chemotherapeutic agent is localized to tumor site.

Injection of contrast agent into the sinus may help to delineate the antral architecture.

US-guided Intervention

1. USG guided FNAC
2. USG guided core biopsy
3. US guided tumor ablation
4. US guided foreign body retrieval
5. Installation of drainage catheter.

Indications of US-guided FNAC/Biopsy

1. It is used for aspiration of small cysts, abscess, fluid collection, tumor, arthrocentesis which are difficult to localize clinically.
2. When the fluid or tumor is close to the vital organs.
3. It is used to choose the shortest and safest route for needle insertion.
4. In bony lesions—bone lesion have been regarded traditionally as a barrier to US imaging. A lytic lesion destroying the cortex, however, can be identified with US as the bright echogenic cortex, which may be accompanied by a soft tissue mass. The defect in the cortex acts like a window through which one can insert a needle under US guidance for the bone marrow aspiration and cytological examination.

US is an ideal way to guide a needle because the steel reflects ultrasound and can therefore be clearly followed as it enters the body. However, it is possible for only part of the needle to show. This can happen if front portion of the needle leaves the scanning plane and becomes invisible. The apparent tip is then actually the point at which the leaves the scanning plane and is not the actual tip of the needle. It may cause damage by puncturing the wrong tissues (Fig. 15.22).

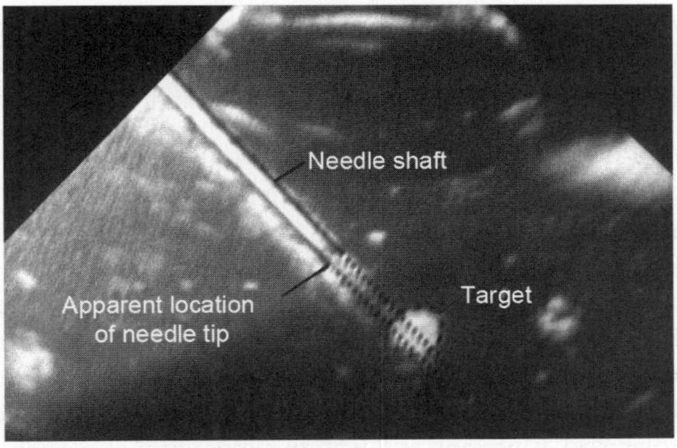

Fig. 15.22: USG guided FNAC, showing apparent location of needle in relation to target

Advantages of US-guided FNAC

1. Allows monitering of the procedure at all times
2. Control the intervention
3. Increses accuracy
4. Safety of procedure.

Disadvantage

It is good in determining the outline of structure but not necessarily their content.

US-guided Tumor Ablation

Direct injection of tumor with either a toxic substance (ethanol) or an immunotherapeutics agent (gene therapy).

A case report regarding the retrieval of minor salivary gland sialoliths of upper lip with real time, US-guided technique.

Indication

1. For placement of plastic probe
2. Monitor the tissue destruction. Tissue become hypoechoic because of gas bubbles.

Advantages of US-guided intervention are increased accuracy and safety of procedure.

Alteration to USG-guided tumor ablation is fluoroscopy and CT guided.

US-guided Foreign Body Retrieval

US is very useful in identifying and localizing radiolucent soft tissue foreign bodies. A foreign body appears as a hyperechoic lesion surrounded by hypoechoic halo thought to represent the inflammatory reaction.

Echocardiography (echo): It is the application of ultrasound to study the anatomy and function of heart. There are different cardiac imaging modalities like ventricular angiograms, angiography, digital subtraction angiography, CT, MRI, ECG, etc.

All above techniques have potential of providing estimates of cardiac size and function but all have limitations, i.e. they are invasive, require IV contrast media and do not provide beat-to-beat information. Echo is an inexpensive, noninvasive technique that provides beat-to-beat information about cardiac size, functions and wall thickness and also enables direct visualization of the cardiac valves which can be assessed qualitatively and quantitatively.

Different Echo techniques— Real time echo
Two-dimensional echo
Doppler cardiography

Echo generally is performed by using a small foot print sector scan. Access to heart taken through intercostals space.

US Biomicroscopy

Using the frequencies of 40–50 MHz imaging of the living tissues can be done at microscopic resolution supplying information previously available from biopsies. Using these system atrial and ventricular contractions have been imaged as early as 9th to 10th day of embryonic development.

Hybrid Arrays

These are formed by coupling piezoelectric material to a microchip detector.

Elastography

Detection of changes in tissue elasticity. Localized changes in tissue elasticity or stiffness are well recognized signs of disease and may provide the earliest indication of abnormality. For example, in tumors of breast and prostate.

Therapeutic US

Low intensity US has been shown to provide a therapeutic benefit in RAS. It accelerates wound healing, decreases number of lesions. The mechanism underlying is the modification of the inflammatory response.

16 Basic Principles of Magnetic Resonance Imaging

HISTORY

Bloch and Purcell described the phenomenon of magnetic resonance imaging (MRI) independently and simultaneously in 1946, During the 1950 and -1960s *Eicik Odeblad*, a Swedish Physicist and Gynecologist studied the proton magnetic resonance properties of human erythrocytes, cervical mucus, myometrium, human milk, saliva and gingival mucosa and fluid of eye. *Mans- Field and Maudstey, Damadian et al and Hinshaw et al* first published human in vivo images in 1977. *Hawkes* first demonstrated the multiplanar facility of MRt in 1980 that reported first time, the demonstration of intracranial pathology by MRI.

Damadian made an important contribution when he observed that the relaxation time of proton within malignant tissue were longer then those of normal tissue.

Dr Damadian received the National Medal of Technology in July 15 1988. *Peter Mans flied* was honored with Noble Prize on 10th December 2003 for his contribution in the flied of diagnostic radiology.

INTRODUCTION

Basic principle of MRI is "bloch equation". Atomic nucleus with an odd number of protons or neutrons is spinning like tops. As a result of the spinning they generate a magnetic field called as magnetic moment (Fig. 16.1A).

MRI is latest noninvasive imaging modality that uses electrical signals generated from the responses of hydrogen nuclei (proton) to a strong magnetic field and radiowaves/radiofrequency pulses to produce an image to allow specialists to explore the inner working of human body, to detect and define the differences between healthy and diseased tissue without the use of X-ray. It enables the radiologist to view, slices of the body cut in different planes increasing the diagnostic ability. The nucleus of the hydrogen atom has just one proton and no neutron with highest sensitivity to magnetic field and are constantly turning around on an axis (Fig. 16.1B).

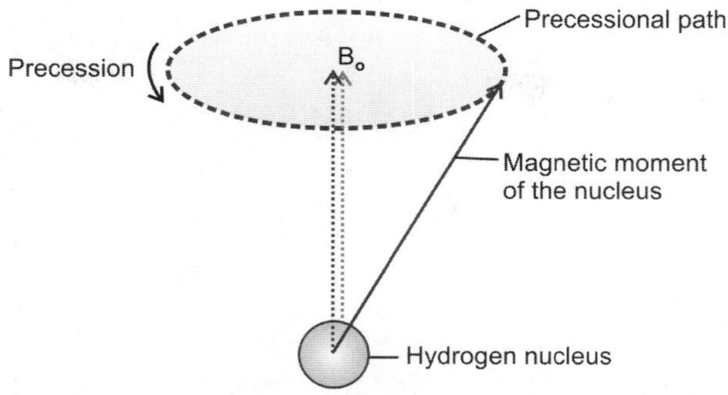

Fig. 16.1A: Precession—magnetic movement of the nucleus

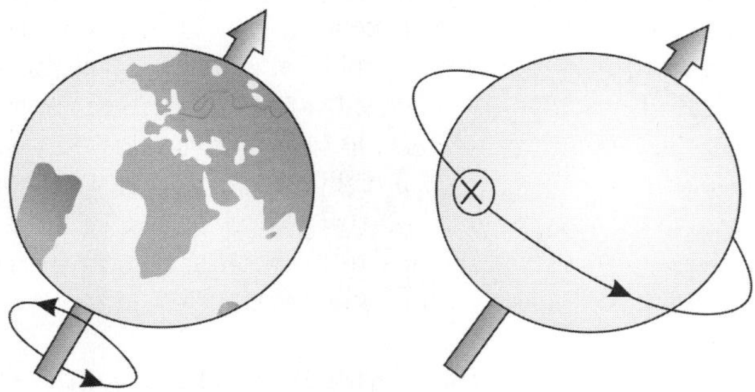

Fig. 16.1B: Protons are constantly turning around on an axis and have their own magnetic field

Principle

The human body is chemical composition of several elements, such as hydrogen, carbon, nitrogen, sodium, phosphorus, potassium, etc. in various chemical combinations. The magnetic properties of the protons of these elements have been utilized to produce magnetic resonance signals and images (Fig. 16.2).

When a patient is placed in the strong magnetic field in the MRI scanner, the hydrogen nucleus in the body, align with applied external magnetic field when exposed to short burst of radio frequency (RF) pulses (Fig. 16.3).

The hydrogen nuclei in the patient's body absorb its energy and then generate MR signal. This process of absorbing energy is known as magnetic resonance. It forms the basics of MR imaging.

Hydrogen nuclei (with single proton) in the absence of external interference are in random motion and their magnetic moment cancel each

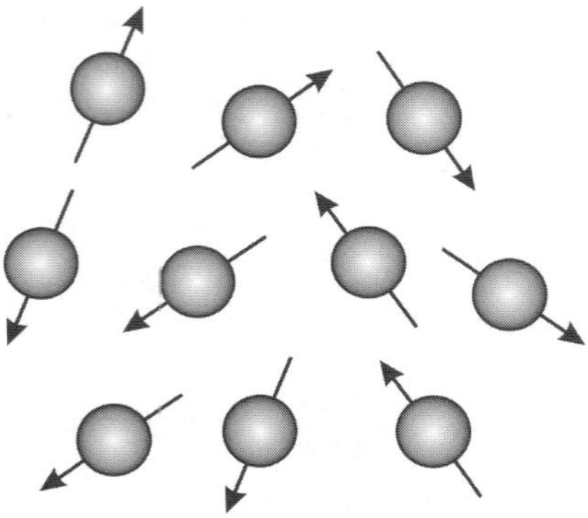

Fig. 16.2: Various MR active nuclei with their atomic number with linear alignment

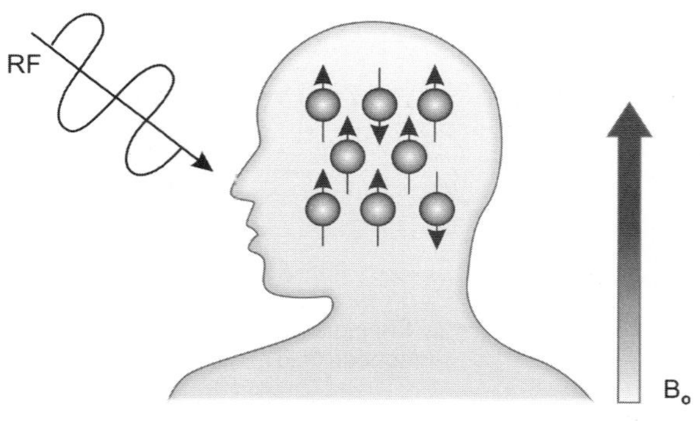

Fig. 16.3: Alignment of body hydrogen nucleus in strong magnetic field

other resulting in overall zero magnetization. When the patient is placed inside the magnetic field, the hydrogen nuclei (proton) in the body get aligned in proper orientation and this leads to the patient being magnetized which in turn emits signals which are captured by the receiver and after a series of processing, transformation result in the formation of images on the screen (Figs 16.4A and B).

Example: When the tissue is subjected to a strong magnetic field the magnetic moments of the tissue will orient with the static magnetic field. However energy in forms of RF is added to this system. The nuclear magnets that are aligned with the magnetic field will flip 90° to 180° (depending on duration and amplitude of the RF) and became misaligned with the field. The nuclei of each species of atom that has a magnet moment has a unique frequency that will cause them to tip in the static magnet field. This is called as the Larmor or NMR frequency (Figs 16.5A to C).

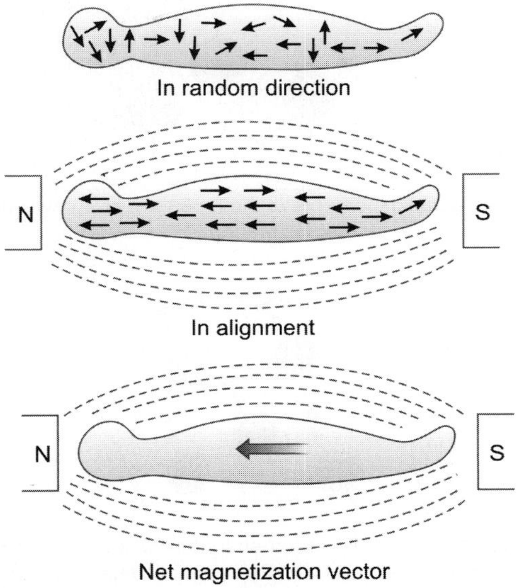

Fig. 16.4A: The patient is placed in the powerful magnetic system

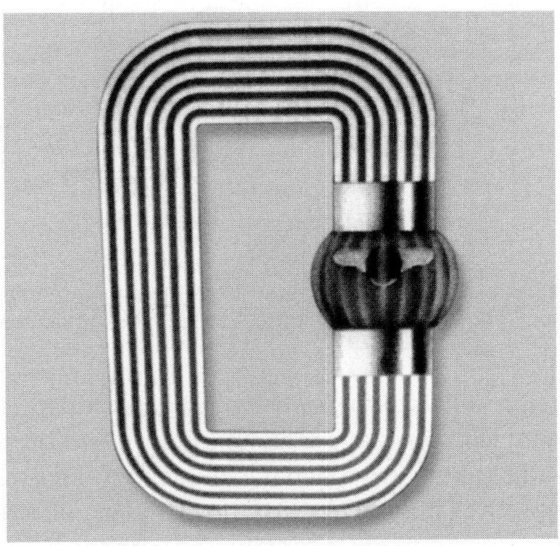

Fig. 16.4B: Alignment of hydrogen protons in human body

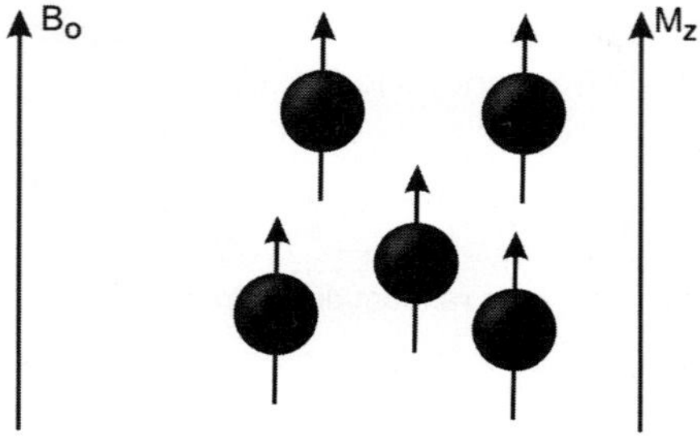

Fig. 16.5A: The magnetic moments of the hydrogen proton will orient with the static magnetic

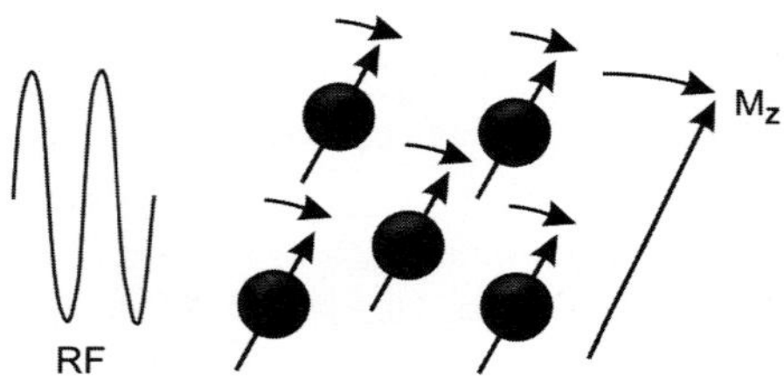

Fig. 16.5B: Energy in forms of RF is added to this system will change the nuclear magnets that are aligned with the magnetic field to 90° to 180°

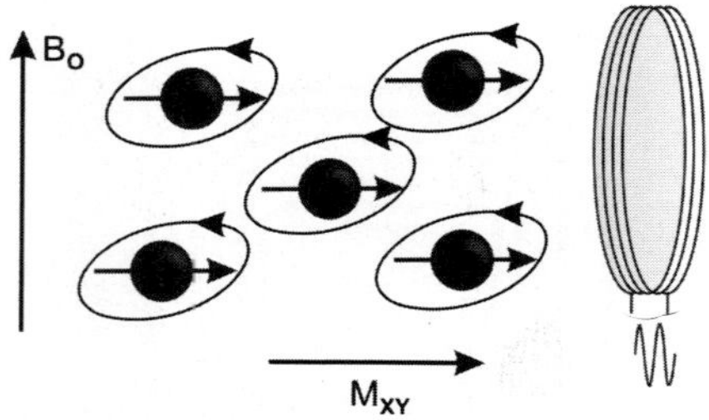

Fig. 16.5C: The nucleus of each species of atom that has a magnet moment has a unique frequency that will cause them to tip in the static magnet field

When the radio signals terminated the nuclear magnets release and flip back in alignment with the static magnetic field. When these nuclei relax they transmit radio signals (RF) that has a frequency unique to the element and signals strength that is indicator of the elements relative abundance. From these radio signals image is constructed with the help of computer.

MR Imaging

Basic physical principles:

1. Radiofrequency pulse to perturb steady—state proton magnetization.
2. Transient, small radio signal emitted.
3. Spatial encoding with magnetic field gradients.
4. Image map of MR signal strength.

The image is generated by four factors:

A. Proton density.
B. T1 relaxation times.
C. T2 relaxation times.
D. Flow.

Proton density is the concentration of protons in the tissue in the form of water and macromolecules (proteins, fat, etc.).

T1 related to energy transfer as a result of thermal interaction between the nuclei and their local environment. Spin lattice or longitudely relaxation time the characteristic time constant for spine to tend to align them with the external magnetic field. T1 of diseased and damaged tissue is longer then for corresponding healthy tissue (Fig. 16.6A).

T2 relates to exchange of energy between nuclei. Spin or transverse relaxation time the characteristic time constant for loss of phase of coherence among spins oriented at an angle to the main magnetic field owing to interactions between the spins. T2 never exceeds T1 (Fig. 16.6B).

The T1 and T2 relaxation times define the way that the protons revert back to their resting states after the initial RF pulse.

Both of these parameters are distinct processes that vary with the relative health of the tissues. The most common effect of flow is loss of signal from rapidly flowing arterial blood.

An MR system consists of the following components:

1. A large magnet to generate the magnetic field.
2. Shim coils to make the magnetic field as homogeneous as possible.
3. A radiofrequency (F) coil to transmit a radio signal into the body part being imaged.
4. A receiver coil to detect the returning radio signals.
5. Gradient coils to provide spatial localization of the signals.
6. A computer to reconstruct the radio signals into the final image (Fig. 16.7).

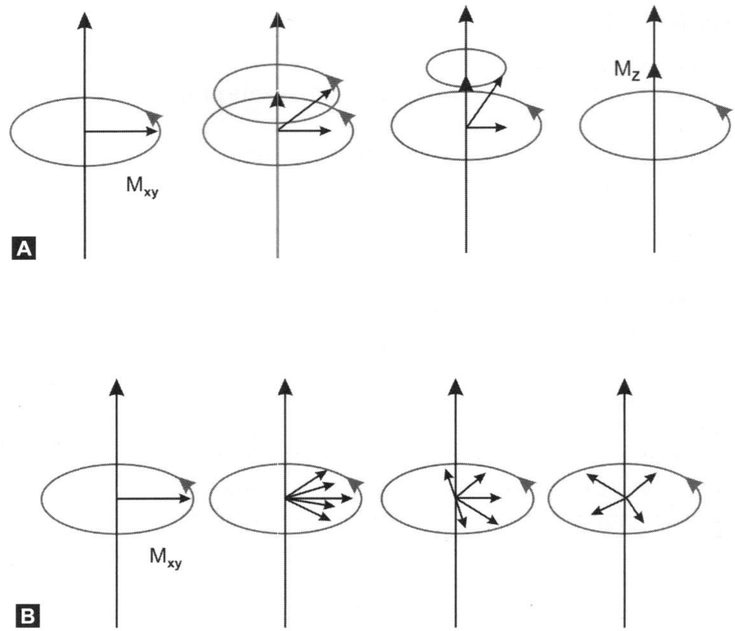

Figs 16.6A and B: Longitude and transverse movement after release of RF wave

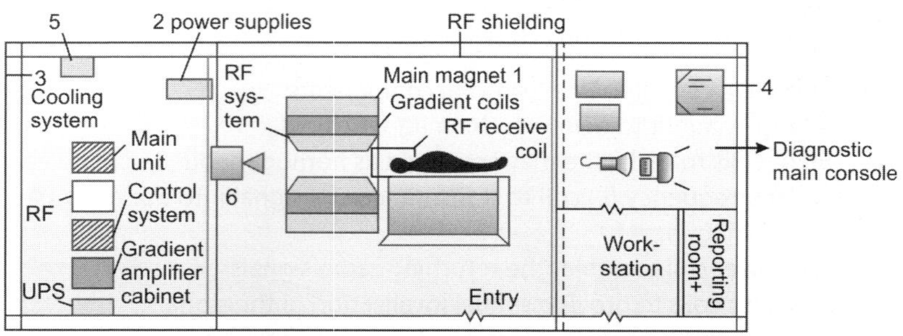

Fig. 16.7: Component of MR system

Magnet

The homogeneous magnetic field required for MR imaging, is generated by a strong magnet, there are three types of magnet are available:

1. Permanent magnets.
2. Electromagnets.
3. Superconducting magnets.

Permanent magnets are:

a. Simple and cheap to run.
b. Extremely heavy.
c. Do not generate high field (Fig. 16.8A).

Electromagnets or Resistive Magnets

a. Magnetic field is generated by an electric current flowing through a coil.
b. Required high electric and cooling system.
c. Difficult to raised more than 1.5 T (Fig. 16.8B).

Superconducting Magnets

a. These are also electromagnets, made of materials with no electric resistance when placed at a temperature closed to absolute zero.
b. They consume no power and allow stable and very high magnetic field.
c. They are more commonly used (Fig. 16.8C).

Coils

Following types of coils are most commonly used for MR imaging:

1. Volume coils: Head/body coil, are both transmit and receive radiofrequency (RF) pulses and called —transceivers. And is fixed inside the magnet
2. Surface/local coils:
   a. Are place closed to the region of interest. Used for imaging the structure near to the skin surface.
   b. Help to improve the signal to noise ratio (SNR).
   c. They only receive the signal.

Phased Array Coil

a. It consists of multiple coils and is receiver only.
b. It is used for larger areas.

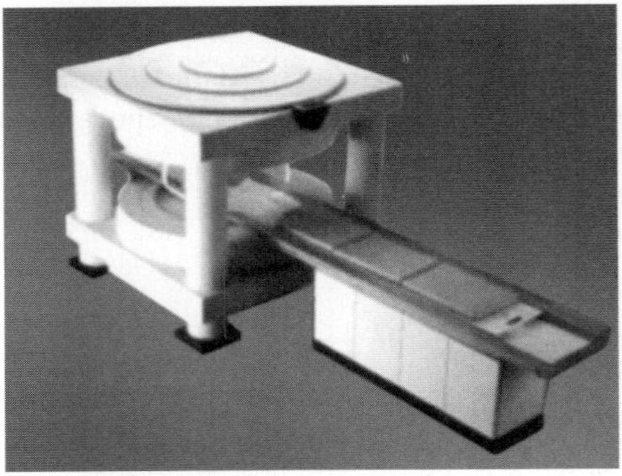

Fig. 16.8A: Permanent magnets

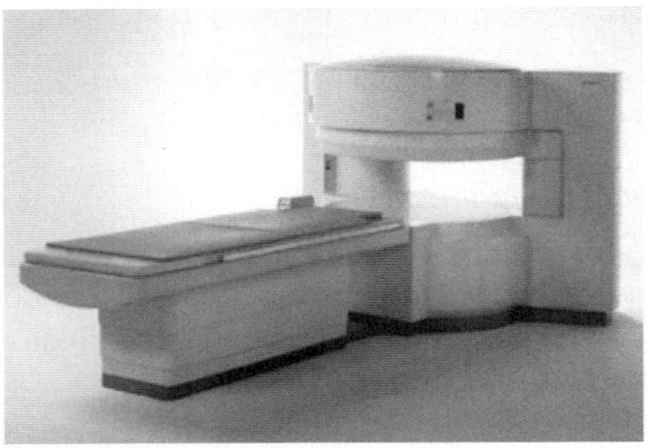

Fig. 16.8B: Electromagnets or resistive magnets

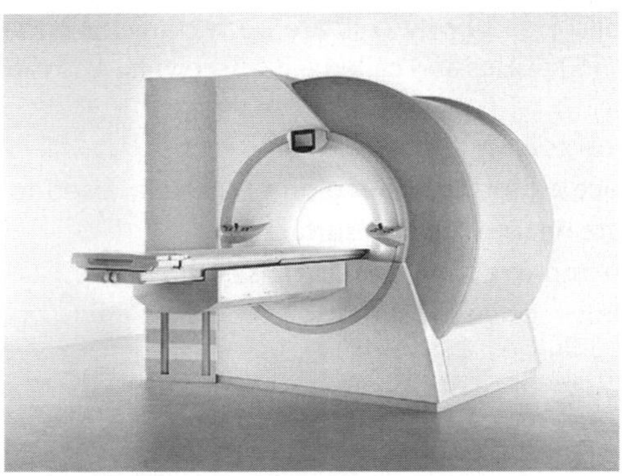

Fig. 16.8C: Superconducting magnets

Gradient Coils

Are the special coils varying the strength of the magnetic field, frequency and phase of the electromagnetic wave in the transverse and longitudinal planes?

Provide spatial localization of the sign (Figs 16.9A to F).

Shielding

The MR signal is relatively weak. Hence, small external RF interferences can significantly degrade the image quality. As a result, imaging room must be shielded from external sources of RF energy. RF shielding will be done into the side wall, floor and ceiling.

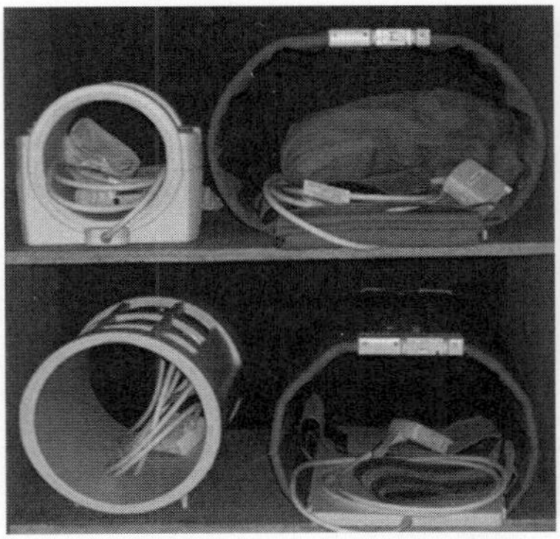

Fig. 16.9A: Various coils use for MRI

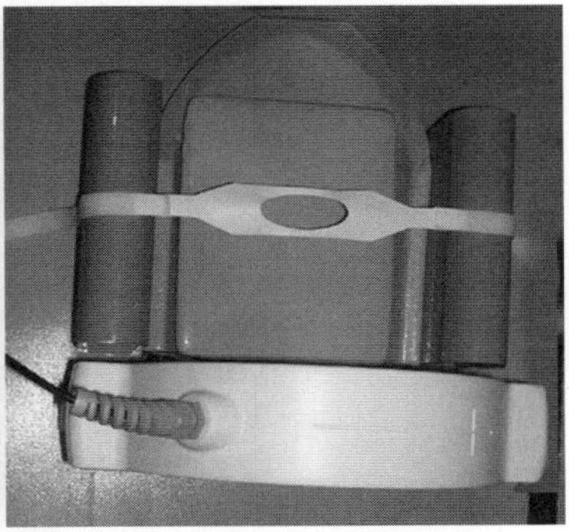

Fig. 16.9B: Head coil

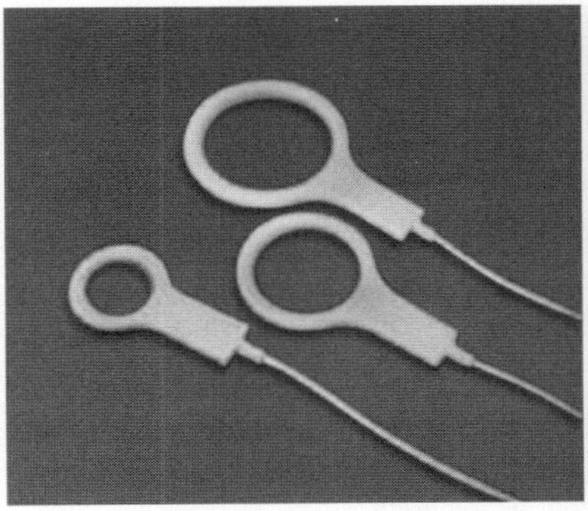

Fig. 16.9C: General purpose flexible MRI coil

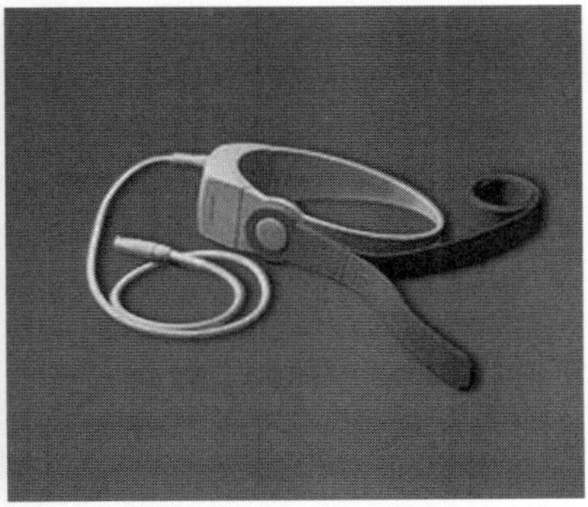

Fig. 16.9D: Shoulder coil

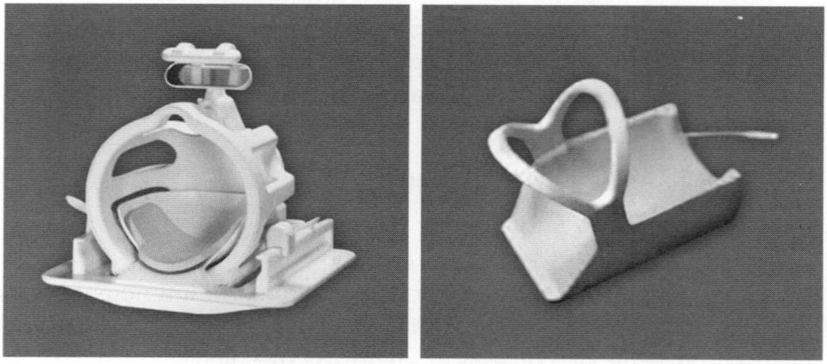

Fig. 16.9E: Phased array coil

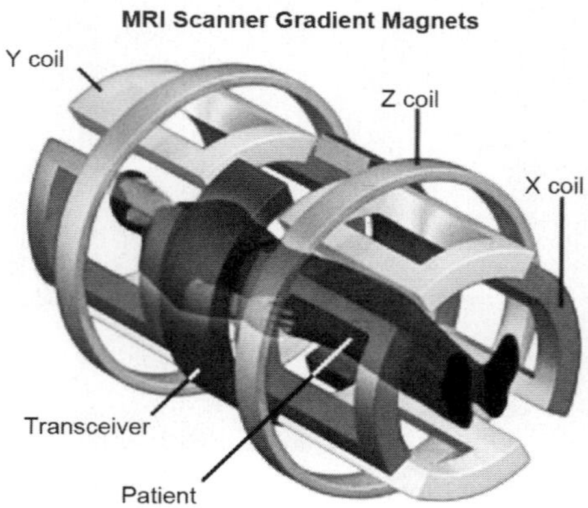

Fig. 16.9F: Gradient coils

Better homogeneity can be achieved by electrical and mechanical adjustments by a process known as shimming may be active shimming or passive shimming. In active shimming several shim coils are attached to shim tube, while in passive shimming small iron plates are attached to magnet.

Camera

The MR images are exposed on X-ray film with the laser camera connected to the MRI system.

Documentation

According to tasks involved, computed data and reconstructed images are stored either in: A fixed storage medium—Magnetic Hard Disks or

A removable storage medium—Magneto Optical Disks,

The contrast on the MR image can be manipulated by changing the pulse sequence parameters.

A pulse sequence sets the specific number, strength, and timing of the RF and gradient pulses.

The two most important parameters are the repetition time (TR) and the echo time (TE).

The TR is the time between consecutive 90° RF pulse. The TE is the time between the initial 90° RF pulse and the echo.

Spin-echo pulse sequence

Single-echo T1-weighted (Figs 16.10A and B).

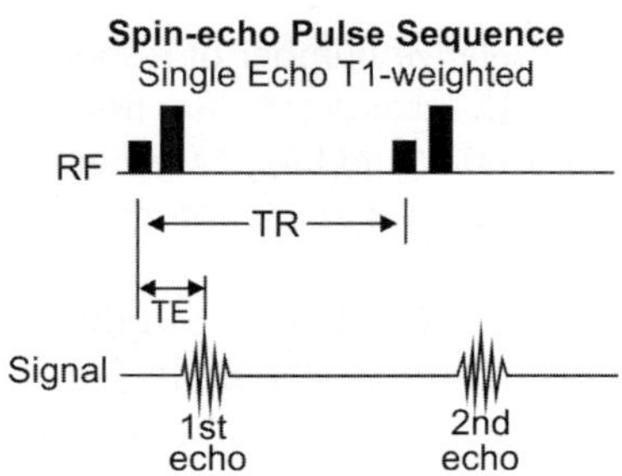

Fig. 16.10A: Single-echo T1-weighted

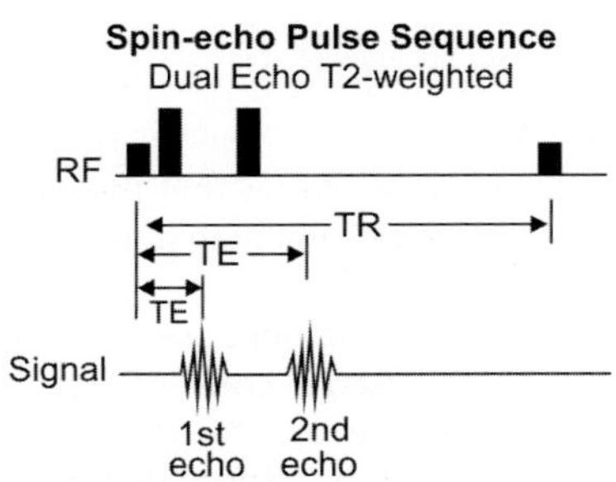

Fig. 16.10B: Dual-echo T2-weighted

The most common pulse sequences are the T1-weighted and T2-weighted spin-echo sequences.

The T1-weighted sequence uses a short TR and short TE (TR <1000 msec, TE < 30 msec).

The T2-weighted sequence uses a long TR and long TE (TR >2000 msec, TE > 80 msec). The T2-weighted sequence can be employed as a dual-echo sequence.

The first or shorter echo (TE < 30 msec) is proton density (PD) weighted or a mixture of Tl and T2. This image is very helpful for evaluating periventricular pathology, such as multiple sclerosis, because the hyperintense plaques are contrasted against the lower signal CSF. More recently, the FLAIR (Fluid Attenuated Inversion Recovery) sequence has replaced the PD image. FLAIR images are:

- T2-weighted with the CSF signal suppressed.
- The TR, matrix size and NEX are the only parameters that affect scan time. Increasing any one of these parameters increases the minimum scan time.
- The spin density or relative number of resonating protons per unit volume is also parameter that determines tissue contrast.
- High spin density, short T1and long T2 generally contribute to high signal (white) on MR images as seen in the marrow, fat within the condyle and articular eminence.
- Low spin density, long Tl and short T2 contribute to low signal (dark) on MR images as seen in the cortical bone.
- All these parameter can be changed by varying the radiofrequency pulse sequences.

MRI Machines

MRI machines are of two types:

- Open MRI unite (Fig. 16.11)
- Closed MRJ unite (Fig. 16.12).

Open MRI unit have two advantages that they can be used for claustrophobic patient, and they provide imaging guidance—for interventional procedures.

Open unit image the patient in larger bore or C-shaped magnets rather than the closed narrow tunnel used in conventional units, these magnets are weaker (0.1–0.3 Tesla) then the closed units.

Close MRI unit are the high field strength unites (0.3–3 Tesla) generally offer more esthetic and diagnostic images then open units.

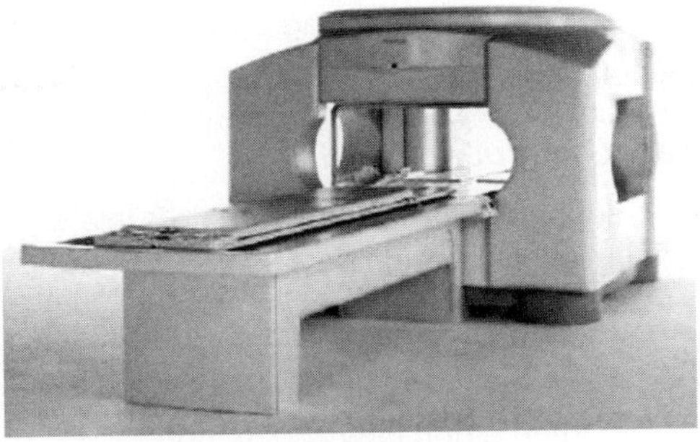

Fig. 16.11: Open MR unite

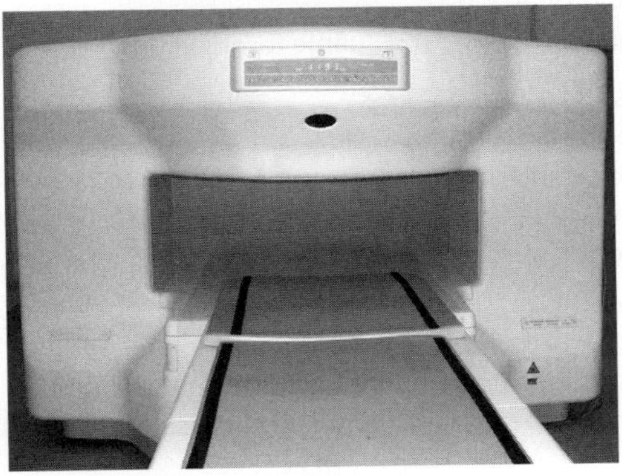

Fig. 16.12: Close MR unite

Imaging Sequences

There are two popular imaging sequences:

- Spin echo (SE)
- Gradient recalled echo (GRE).

Spin-echo sequences allow the examiner to use both T1and T2 magnetic resonance imagings. The repetition time (TR) and echo time (TE) are parameters controlled by the operator and they can be used in relation to the T1 and T2 values in the tissues to optamize image contrast and resolution, this process called weighting.

1. A long TR and short TE produce proton density weighting.
2. A short TR and short TE produce Tl-weighting, and is best for examining the normal temporomandibular joint (TMJ).
3. A long TR and long TE produce T2-weighting and best for detecting inflammations and effusion of the joint.

Spin-echo uses an initial 90° flip angle with subsequently refocusing RF pulse of 180°.

Gradient-recalled Sequences (GREs)

- Very short TRs are possible as RF pulse angle is less then 90°.
- Reducing the image acquisition time.
- Frequently used for TMJ in the pseudodynamic (cine) fashion.
- Fast images can be obtained (for each image) 25 second required.
- Signal to noise ratio decreased causes inferior images.
- It is useful for imaging blood flow and hemorrhage.

Normal MRI Anatomy of TMJ:

T1-wight image are the most valuable for depicting normal TMJ anatomy.

These images show the:

- Cortical bone as dark to black
- Articular disk and dense fascia—more dark to gray
- Normal muscles—gray
- Fat and Bone marrow—white.

The fascial sheaths that cover the pterygoid muscles appears white or lighter gray then muscles.

The osseous TMJ components include the mandibular condyle, the glenoid fossa and the articular eminence; these appear white with black outline.

Osseous boundaries include the anterior slope of the articular eminence, the tympanic portion of temporal bone posteriorly.

The roots of the zygomatic arch laterally.

Temporal process medially.

When reviewing an MR image, the easiest way to determine which pulse sequence was used, or the "weighting" of the image, is to look at the cerebrospinal fluid (CSF).

If the CSF is bright (high signal), then it must be a T2-weighted imaged. If the CSF is dark, it is a Tl-weighted image.

MR Signal Intensities:

	T2WI	*PD/FLAIR*	*T1WI*
Solid mass	Bright	Bright	Dark
Cyst	Bright	Dark	Dark
Subacute blood	Bright	Bright	Bright
Acute and chronic	Dark	Dark	Gray
blood—fat	Dark	Bright	Bright

Although the axial plane is the primary plane for imaging the brain, the multiplanar capability of MR allows one; to select the optimal plane to visualize the anatomy of interest.

Coronal views are good for parasagittal lesions near the vertex and lesions immediately above or below the lateral ventricles, temporal lobes, sella, and internal auditory canals.

The coronal plane can be used as the primary plane of imaging in patients with temporal lobe seizures.

Sagittal views are useful for midline lesions and for the brain stem and cerebellar vermis.

Clinical Indications

Due to its high sensitivity for brain water, MR is generally more sensitive for detecting brain abnormalities during the early stages of disease. For example, in cases of cerebral infarction, close brain tumors or infections, the MR scan will become positive earlier than CT. When early diagnosis is critical for favorable patient outcome, such as in suspected herpes encephalitis, MR is the imaging procedure of choice.

MR is exquisitely sensitive for white matter disease, such as multiple sclerosis. Close progressive multifocal leukoencephalopathy, leukodystrophy, and post-infectious encephalitis. Patients with obvious white matter abnormalities on MR may have an entirely normal CT scan.

Other clinical situations where MR will disclose abnormalities earlier and more definitively are temporal lobe epilepsy, close non-hemorrhagic brain contusions and traumatic shear injuries.

In general, nonenhancing disease processes are much more apparent on MR than CT.

The value of MR for defining congenital malformations is unquestioned.

The multiplanar display of anatomy gives important information about the corpus callosum and posterior fossa structures.

The phenomenon of flow void within arteries on spin-echo images, the high sensitivity for hemorrhage and hemosiderin deposition,

MR angiography gives MR distinct advantages over CT for imaging vascular disease.

Vascular stenosis or occlusions, aneurysms, arteriovenous malformations can be imaged without intravenous contrast media.

In cases of cryptic vascular malformations and cavernous angiomas, where the angiogram and CT scan are often negative, MR may reveal small deposits of hemosiderin from prior small hemorrhages.

Advantages of MRI

- MRI is noninvasive. MRI shows excellent soft tissue contrast.
- Multiplaner imaging is possible.
- No known biological hazard.
- Normal control volunteers can be imaged.
- Blood flow imaging measurement is possible.
- Imaging of tissue in their function.
- Morphology of vascular system can be image (MRI angiography).

Disadvantages of MRI

- Lack of signal from the cortical bone—appears black on MRI
- Limitations of its use in patients with cardiac pacemakers, spinal implants aneurysmal clips or metallic foreign body as these metallic objects interfere with the imaging procedure.
- Reduced patient cooperation due to long imaging time may exhibit motion and result in artifacts.
- It is very expensive and the services are not easily available.
- Many protocol options.
- Correct choice of machine parameters essential.
- Difficult to manage and monitor patients who are critical.

Applications

1. In demyelination diseases.
2. Image of soft tissues without ionizing radiation and contrast media.
3. *Tongue imaging*: Mainly in lingual tumor for definition of boundaries, the degree of vascularity.
4. Salivary gland imaging.
5. In TMJ soft tissue evaluation.

MRI Technique

- Before entering the MRI chamber the patient is advised to remove any jewelry, watch, metal pen, coins, credit card, mobile phones that he/she may be having on his/her body.
- The patient is made to lie down in the supine position for the MRI.
- Imaging is done with a special TMJ coil.
- Surface coil is place around the patient head.
- With the help of laser light longitudinal and transverse plane are adjusted.

- Laser light is put off.
- Patient is put into MRI scanner (Fig. 16.13).
- Ones the patient is ready, MRI room must be closed.
- With the help of console patient details are recorded.
- After recording the patient details selects the area of interest (Figs 16.14A and B).

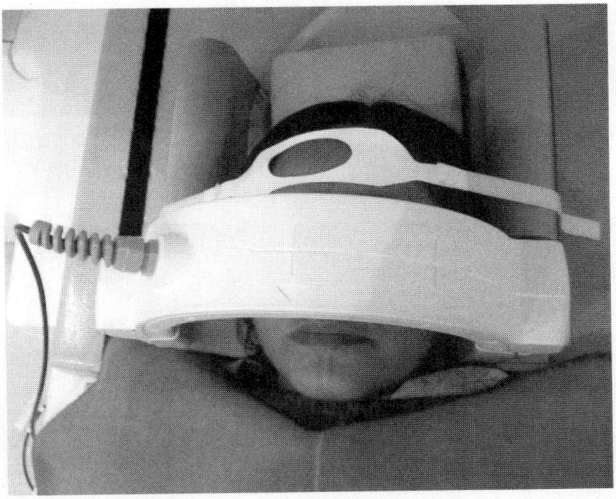

Fig. 16.13: Patient's position with head coil in MRI system

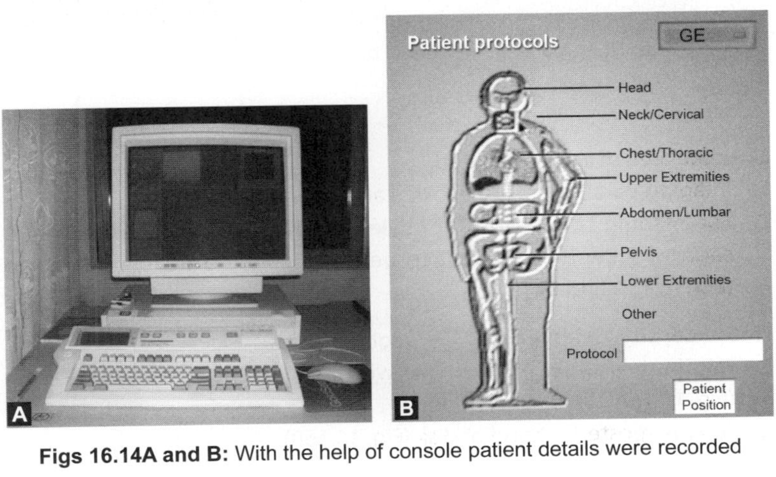

Figs 16.14A and B: With the help of console patient details were recorded

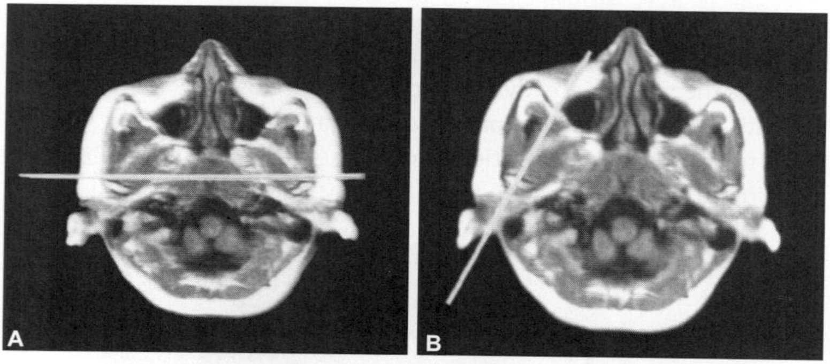

Figs 16.15A and B: (A) Head of condyle is located; (B) To achieve oblique sagittal view lines are place perpendicular to head of condyle

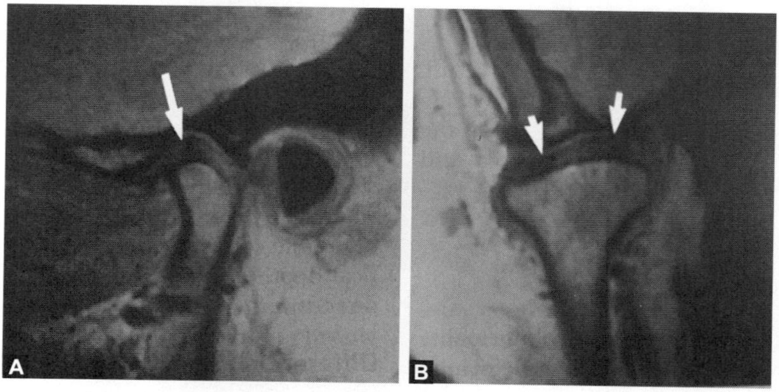

Figs 16.16A and B: MR image of TMJ: Showing articular disc

Ones the area of scan is decided.

- Imaging parameters are decided and selected.
- For imaging TMJ, head of condyle is located and to achieve oblique sagittal view lines are place perpendicular to head of condyle (Fig. 16.15A and B).

Proton density-weighted and T2-weighted

- MR images show normal TMJ with no evidence of joint effusion (Fig. 16.16A).
- Arrow—posterior band of disk (Fig. 16.16B).

Index

Page numbers followed by f to figure respectively

U

V

W

X

Z